$\mathcal{F}irst\ Opinion$

Wholistic Health Care for the 21st Century

by
Barbara Condron
D.M., D.D., B.J.

SOM Publishing
WIndyville, Missouri 65783 U.S.A.

© January, 1998
by the School of Metaphysics No. 100157

Cover Art by Sharka Glet

ISBN: 0-944386-18-0

Library of Congress Catalogue Number pending

PRINTED IN THE UNITED STATES OF AMERICA

If you desire to learn more about the research and teachings in this book, write to School of Metaphysics, National Headquarters, Windyville, Missouri 65783. Or call 417-345-8411.

One may heal with holiness,

one may heal with the law,

one may heal with the knife,

one may heal with herbs,

one may heal with the Holy Word;

amongst all remedies this one is the healing one

that heals with the Holy Word;

this one is that will best drive away

sickness from the body of the faithful.

– Zend Avesta, 6th century B.C.

Foreword

Not long ago, our two-year-old son Hezekiah came running up to me saying, "Mama, heal it."

In his urge to get into the kitchen as quick as possible, he had forgotten to remember to look with his mind before moving his body. As a result he had run into the dining room table, "bump head" as he would say.

Having seen the collision, I knew his reaction was more shock than physical damage. I immediately embraced him, and while quietly asking him what happened I directed healing energy to his mind and body. Asking Hezekiah questions gave him a point of focus, moving his mind from the injury to his natural excitement for learning how to communicate. Once he was involved in describing his experience, I was free to restore his mental and emotional health, coalescing his scattered thoughts and refreshing depleted energies. Then I mentally assessed any physical harm and responded accordingly, directing healing energy to tissue, nerves and blood vessels in the affected area. Within seconds Hezekiah was on his way again.

Hezekiah is learning. He isn't learning about drugstores, children's aspirin, or doctors and hospitals. He is learning that he possesses an abundant capacity for health, and that the power for perpetual well-being is always with him. Hezekiah knows that mama and daddy can heal. He has felt the results of our healing many times. And—as he has demonstrated with his stuffed animal toys, "Heal bunny!"—he naturally believes he too can heal. Daily my husband and I teach him what we have learned about the nature of consciousness. He is learning that the power to move, to speak, to sing, to comprehend, comes from within and so does the capacity to heal. Hezekiah is learning the most basic of Universal Truths: *thought is cause.*

Each of us sees the world as we are taught to live it. In every culture, most of this comes from parents and others in the home environment. What we learn early in life does shape the way we think. This is when we learn to rely upon either supernatural intervention or physical authority in times of health crisis. Childhood is where we live with patterns of sound minds and resilient bodies, or unstable minds and weakened bodies. This is where we begin to imitate what we see causing others' beliefs to become our own. What we know arises from the experiences first imaged in our minds.

Within this ancient and universal truth – *thought is cause and the physical is its manifest likeness* – is the key to health and well-being. The concept is purely fundamental, so simple that a two-year-old can grasp it, so straightforward that the worldly-wise often miss it.

This truth operates throughout our universe. It shows no favoritism. It does not matter where you live on the planet, who your parents are, what your income is, or even the level of your education or religious preference. It doesn't even matter whether you are aware of this truth in your life or not, thought is cause. Thought is where wellness or illness begins, where prosperity or poverty begins, where accord or strife begins, companionship or loneliness. It is the beginning, and all else follows accordingly. As the master teacher Jesus of Nazareth taught, "Seek ye first the kingdom of Heaven and all else will be given unto you."

Your power to heal arises from the Source of creation, whatever you consider It to be. In the 1800's Mary Baker Eddy, founder of Christian Science, said, "We classify disease as error, which nothing but Truth or Mind can heal, and this Mind must be divine, not human." Her words are as true now as they were a hundred or even a thousand years ago.

With all the scientific and technological discoveries of this century Mankind, as never before, is wrestling with His divinely inherent potential for wholeness. Science enables us to experiment as creators. Medical advances extend man's power to know the circumstances and time of his physical birth and of his physical death, introducing him to the clairvoyant powers attributed to the Creator. More and more Man is aware of his power to determine the conditions of life and death, realms previously left in the care of a Supreme Being. Yet too often the purpose for Man's existence escapes him because he has yet to give the respect, dignity, responsibility, and credit to the power of thought as the origin for all physical manifestations. The mind can slay and the mind can heal.

One thing is certain, we must continue to be open-minded, we must continue to learn, or we are destined to manifest only what we were taught as children. The world continues to change, whether its inhabitants elect to or not. The universe is constantly evolving, whether Humankind is transformed or not. We must admit that any knowledge that aids us to grow, to reach, to learn, to discover, to understand, is invaluable. The wisdom which arises from putting that knowledge into practice is that much more desirable.

The faculty and students of the School of Metaphysics are courting this enlightened wisdom. During the past quarter century, research into the nature of consciousness and the Universal Laws governing creation has reaped phenomenal insights. One of the most gratifying developments of our studies is the unifying of science and religion, philosophy and discipline, thought and action, as a means of creating wholeness in Self.

For many this is quite a controversial area. Scientists and theologians are often at odds. Even amongst themselves these people are often at odds, after all when one begins arguing to be right one has lost sight of the pursuit for truth.

What we are discovering is how Universal Law demonstrates itself throughout our lives. This common ground transcends all physical differences offering hope, challenge, and promise to Humankind. We are dedicated to sharing the benefits of our research with the world. I believe our findings are timely and will help accelerate humanity's progression, as individuals and as a species, toward a profound spirituality.

As Western medical pioneer Jonas Salk observed, "The fitness of the future is wisdom." What is worthy of noting is the means by which most will come to this soundness of mind. It is true that for most people the desire alone for peace of mind is not a sufficient motivating force for healthy change in attitude and lifestyle. However, panicked need for quality care can provide the call to action that will be heeded. People want the security of knowing the best care is available and affordable. And with today's Western allopathic medicine both are becoming scarce.

As a result, soon economics will be the reason for people developing their full potential – mentally and spiritually as well as physically. Practically speaking, the pressure to reduce the use of expensive, conventional technologies such as magnetic resonance imaging (MRI) is even now opening the door to new forms of medical diagnosis. Speaking to a convention of the Parapsychological Association, Larry Burk, a radiologist at Durham University Medical School, said that medical intuitives may be able to provide comparably useful information for screening purposes while allowing the most cost effective use of hi-tech diagnostic methods. He called for empirical studies comparing the results produced by sensitives with known findings from x-rays.

This is the kind of research the School of Metaphysics pursues; in fact our Intuitive Health Analysis is like a MRI accomplished with the highly disciplined and attuned mind instead of a machine. A growing number of health practictioners, from physicians to chiropractors to naturopaths, consider these analyses a welcome addition to the treatment of their patients. The information revealed in a reading helps them to provide quality health care to the whole person. Others, like the Shealy Institute, refer their patients to us because we provide an intuitive analysis, a diagnosis they do not have available. It seems with each passing year of this last century, care from a family doctor who knows you and your family declined as technology and insurance escalated. The Intuitive Health Analysis empowers health practitioners to once again be a profound healing influence.

Part of the untapped potential of each human being is the vast frontier of intuitive knowledge and skill. It is the product of a more familiar ability, reasoning. Those familiar with the School of Metaphysics' course of study know that the spiritual disciplines and mental exercises presented are intended to stimulate and cultivate these areas. In fact the second series of lessons focus upon the consciously aware development of intuitive sensitivity.

The possibilities of intuitive knowledge as it is applied to the well-being of an individual, has been one of the cornerstones in our research for a quarter of a century. This is particularly true with the Intuitive Health Analyses. These analyses, conducted by trained teams of a reader and a conductor, are a report of intuitively perceived disorders in mind and body. Time and again our findings have been seconded by hi-tech diagnoses. And time and again the health analyses reveal what allopathic medicine as yet cannot.

Intuitive Health Analyses are truly astounding for they offer invaluable information about the state of mind as well as the state of the body. Throughout the 1900's, conventional Western medicine began to admit the importance of a patient's frame of mind in recovery and even in susceptibility to illness. What is dawning now will mature in the coming centuries. Eventually the direct connection between ways of thinking and the health or illness of the physical body will become commonly accepted. We will move beyond the outer perimeters of being into the causal realms within each of us. Eventually we will embrace the powers inherent in our consciousness. We will be healers and our children will learn to be also. Intuitive knowledge will become more commonplace as we seek to understand ourselves and each other, to ensure good health, and to control our destiny. The School of Metaphysics responds to all of these universal needs. We are dedicated to the wholistic education and services that promote spiritual well-being and wholistic health. You are about to learn much of what we have discovered. I trust it will motivate you to take control of your health, teach you new ways to be healthy, and inspire you to fulfill your purpose for being here. Thank you for supporting our work and sharing it with others.

Barbara Condron
College of Metaphysics
1997

When health is absent,

wisdom cannot reveal itself,

art cannot become manifest,

strength cannot be exerted,

wealth is useless and reason is powerless.

– Herophilus, 300 B.C.

To keep the body in good health is a duty,

for otherwise we shall not be able

to trim the lamp of wisdom,

and keep our mind strong and clear.

Water surrounds the lotus flower, and does not wet its petals.

–Gautama the Buddha
Sermon at Benares, 5th century B.C.

Table of Contents

*L*ook to your health;

and if you have it, praise God,

and value it next to a good conscience;

for health is the second blessing that we mortals are capable of;

a blessing that money cannot buy.

— Izaak Walton, The Compleat Angler 1635

A 21st Century Miracle

Marie is a woman you would do well to know for in the knowing your hopes are confirmed and your dreams uplifted. Marie is a 21st century miracle.

Approaching seventy, she has lived a varied and full life, often facing physical hardship. From shingles at age four to a mild heart attack in her mid-thirties to her more recent health challenges, she has met them all with supernatural faith and courage. She is an inspiration to everyone she meets and anyone who knows her story.

I have known Marie all my life. She is my mother. I want to tell you part of her story for she is truly a testimony to the human potential for resurrection.

My mother's recent trials began sixteen years ago when her mother went to sleep and never awoke. I remember Marie telling me she believed her mother had gone so quickly because her father had learned he had prostate cancer. It was in these small ways that I first learned of the power of thought.

Marie knew well the bond between her parents. Years of shared experience had entwined their hearts and forged a commitment that transcended anything on this earth. Without doubt my mother knew her mother did not want to live without her husband. It was not a matter of wanting to die, it was a matter of how she wanted to live. To my grandmother dying meant the fulfillment of a spiritual promise, joining God in Heaven; a place where she could wait for her husband to join her.

Her death was harder on my grandfather than any of us could have imagined. For months, he would dissolve into tears as memories clouded his thinking. My mother began to care for him, trying to fill some of the void in his life. The constant emotional exhaustion left little energy for his body, and as his health began a slow descent his expectations escalated. Mother's daily visits extended into a permanent live-in situation.

Marie spent the next eight years caring for her father. At first it was running errands, shopping, and paying bills. Then as the disease, and medical treatments, progressed my grandfather became more and more dependent on her for care. Daily tasks of living that were at one time taken for granted now became major trials requiring assistance.

Mother later told me it was like taking care of a baby again, except this time the baby was often physically too large for her to manage. In the final months, when radiation treatments left his right arm useless, mother would cut meat for him and help him bathe. She devoted all of her time, all of her energy, all of her concern, all of her love to her father. He was the center of her universe. Although complaints from her were rare, caring for her father was an enormous physical drain, as well as a mental and emotional strain that would eventually take its toll.

In the fall of 1990, grandfather died. He had been hospitalized for weeks, so the passing was not at all sudden. For mother it was a relief as much as a sorrow, a freedom as much as a loss, a blessing as well as a curse. For the first time in almost a decade, Marie was on her own. No one to dress or feed or care for throughout the day. No more half-alert nights listening for a call for help. At last mother could do all those things she had been putting off.

But there were some problems. Things were not turning out as she had planned. The husband she had left years before had married someone else. Communication between mother and me, her only child, had grown strained in those years, and then existent only when I initiated it. Friendships that were once strong had long since withered from lack of attention. Rebuilding her life required a greater investment than she expected and as it turned out more energy than she had to give. The mental and emotional toll of these changes became apparent within months.

The focal point of her life had left taking much of her life force with him. Within a year following her father's death, mother was hospitalized. She had vomited to the point of losing blood and was rushed to the hospital emergency room. An abdominal hernia was diagnosed and an operation performed. While in the hospital, doctors became aware of the toll on her physical body. They suspected significant liver damage, so significant that the doctors in her hometown really didn't feel that they were equipped to be able to respond to her condition. They recommended seeing specialists at Barnes Hospital in St. Louis, three hours away. Uncertain and scared, she agreed.

It was as she was leaving to go to St. Louis that I learned of her ill health through my dad who had heard from a friend that she was hospitalized. I immediately traveled to be with her, staying through most of the three weeks of intensive tests. We had not spent this much time together since I was a teenager. We learned to walk hand in hand, together, while the doctors probed and poked and photographed. Midst the cold machinery and antiseptic aroma of the outer environment, mother and I initiated a time of reconciliation and healing that has served as the foundation for her recovery.

Mending our hearts was indeed serendipitous because the allopathic specialists had very little to offer. These doctors told Marie that she had a one in ten chance of living a year if she did not receive a liver transplant. And that without it she would live no longer than five years.

Although physically ravaged, mother was spiritually strong upon hearing the medical diagnosis. Holding her hand, I told her it was her decision to make and that I would be there for her no matter what she decided. She spoke of her tiredness, feeling that she would not be able to endure the extensive operation. She had not yet recovered from the hernia removal and could not imagine going through a much longer, more difficult procedure. And she didn't want to be in a position to wait, wondering if the doctors would call today to say a liver was available. She knew the constant suspense would wear her down mentally and emotionally. She couldn't afford that. And finally, if she did have the transplant and survived would she have the strength to make the difficult adjustments of the first two years? She didn't believe she did.

The fact that she was sixty years old and that this was a teaching hospital was not lost on her either. She did not want to be someone's guinea pig, however well-intentioned and caring they might be.

I saw her point although from a slightly different angle. After all the tests, this medical recommendation sounded too much like a death threat to me, let us do this or you die. One in ten is just another way of saying there is a ten percent area we – in this case medical science – don't know about. From my varied research and education, I knew there were many, many alternatives that were not even considered in these figures.

Some of those alternatives my mother had taught me as a child. The most profound is the power of prayer. My mother and I share a profound belief in supernatural healing. Our religious upbringing had proven to us time and again that people who are sick can and do instantaneously heal. Both she and I have experienced such healing on more than one occasion. It's called faith healing, divine intervention, psychic healing, spontaneous regeneration, a miracle. The name is not as important as the fact that we have witnessed this power hundreds of times. And when it came time to make her decision it is this faith that led mother to, as she would say, "Leave it in God's hands."

Mother is not a passive person. When she "turns something over to the Lord" she cooperates with it. At the moment mother left Barnes Hospital to come home, she fixed her mind on the goal she continues to image to this day, "I just want to get well." She does what she knows how to do to achieve what she wants and leaves the rest to the Lord. This quality of thought causes the Universal Laws to work on your behalf. And for healing to transpire, those Laws must be called upon.

Marie moved back to her hometown and was hospitalized for several months. Medical care was the least of what she received during this time. She was pampered, just as she had once cared for her father. Her physical needs were met. She could rest and recuperate, rebuilding strength. She began to change in attitude. In time she recovered her "old self" becoming a constant source of joy to doctors, nurses, and other patients. She built lasting friendships with several nurses. She became the light of the hospital, everyone knew her and looked forward to her "daily rounds".

During this time I stayed with her whenever I was free to travel. Our sense of unity was returning to us in a profound way. And family took on a whole new dimension when I introduced her to the man who would become the son she never had. She immediately fell in love with Daniel, and was like a schoolgirl helping select invitations, designs, and dresses for the upcoming wedding.

Now that she had something to look forward to her strength returned. So did her desire and willingness to go home. A year following her "1 in 10 chance of survival" Marie had moved back into her duplex, totally self sufficient.

She is a testimony, not to medical prediction, but to the healing power of faith, love, commitment, and expectation.

Now, six years later, Marie's resurrection continues. She has embraced the new life she is creating. She goes where she wants to go: shopping, visiting, even trips to Florida with friends during the cold Missouri winters. She visits relatives and friends, brightening their day with her special warmth. She is realizing that many, many people appreciate her kindness and need the strength of her faith.

And in return for her generous spirit of giving a long forsaken desire has been resurrected in her life in the form of a thriving grandson. Her eyes glisten and her heart swells as she hears someone call her "Grandma 'Ree'". She is finding avenues for giving that she never imagined before.

Yes, she has given us a couple scares here and there, requiring the kind of immediate surgical attention only modern medicine can provide. And everyone at the hospital remembers her, so she is treated like a queen when she needs their help.

Always quick with a smile and kind word, Marie uplifts the spirit of everyone she meets. To her no one is a stranger for we are all spiritual brothers and sisters, children of God. She is like an angel of the Lord ministering to others just by being who she is. Her life stands as a testimony to the innate power to heal that exists within each of us. For those who know her she is a constant reminder that God helps those who help themselves...and others.

Marie is a testimony to wholistic healing.

She is a perfect example of the innate power to heal that is present within us at all times. Her way of believing, thinking, and acting exemplifies the human capacity for transformation. Her life reveals the kind of changes that must transpire in the spirit, in the mind, and in the body for lost health to be restored.

In terms of her body, Marie takes care of herself. For the most part she eats foods that are easy for her to digest, more fruits and vegetables, less meats and oily foods. She takes vitamin supplements and exercises through her daily activities. She continues to receive medical attention. Marie uses what is available, what modern science provides. She is on medication that helps her to support what her failing liver will no longer provide. She works with her body to cooperate with its condition, she doesn't ask it to do more than it can but always expects it to do more.

Marie sleeps often, she knows she usually feels better after a good rest. The body is a house for the soul. Because of her familiarity with Biblical teachings mother would call it a temple. By "getting out of the way" her body – the genetic code acting in response to Universal Laws – can rejuvenate itself without interference.

Yet Marie is what medical science calls a miracle. She has beaten all the odds. Surpassing their expectations, she astounds her doctors. They know that these physical steps alone would not have extended her life past the fatalistic predictions of 1991. Most are given reason to pause, marveling at the hows and whys that reach beyond what they know from physical science.

Mother is also a testimony to the power of the mind to heal. In the realm of consciousness, Mother's ideas, thoughts, and attitudes have been resurrected. She is a testimony to the undeniable impact of mental (and emotional) well-being upon the health of the physical body.

All those years Marie was caring for her father she had a reason to live. The reason became a compulsion that drove her to exhaustion. The shock of his death left a place in her empty. Her father had consumed her time and energy for almost a decade. In her concern for him she had sacrificed her marriage, estranged her daughter, and allowed friendships to drift. When he died she suddenly found that she no longer had a place to give. Through the years she had replaced one family with another, and when her father died that sense of family went with him. She believed she was alone.

The relevance of the way we think to physical health is increasingly accepted by experts in the field. Moving beyond generalities of "stress" or "pressure", our research into consciousness traces specific thought patterns that can heal or harm. For instance, time and again Intuitive Health Analyses point to *the reason to live* as the attitude that causes the body's liver to perform its function. A purpose for living feeds the liver, providing it with the life-giving energy it needs to perpetuate the vitality of the body. The attitude is not only relevant, it is a point of origin and therefore the key to health or sickness. Resurrect the health-producing attitude and the body is restored. My mother's longevity proves this theory. She has a "new" family, many friends, even more acquaintances. She is active in building a new church and often visits the elderly or sick. She knows she is needed, and she is happy to give. Resurrecting her consciousness to create another reason to live has empowered Mother and it has enabled her liver to rejuvenate.

Mother is a testimony to spirit, the indomitable spirit that each of us possesses. The will to live, the desire to give, the reaching toward wholeness. She is very aware of existences beyond that of the physical body and its five senses. She knows there is more to man than the flesh, and she communes with her Maker every day through prayer. What she may not be able to accomplish, she is certain that God can. This steadfast belief motivates her to greater good. She is constantly proving and improving herself to be worthy of receiving what she requests.

Indeed Marie's faith influences the calibre of her thinking. It buoys her attitude when she might be inclined to sink into pessimism. It supports her when the weight of her challenges might seem too much to bear. It cleanses her emotions restoring joy to her life. It replenishes her energy and provides the spark for her desire to give.

Spirit. It was mother's faith in Someone greater than herself that resurrected her consciousness.

Mind. Faith gives her the freedom to imagine, to go beyond others' expectations.

Body. This belief that anything is possible puts her in touch with the Source of the innate power to heal.

Wholeness. Acting upon those beliefs matures them into knowing. And her faith is fulfilled.

This book is dedicated to Marie and to my dad Bill,
who has his own story of life and death struggles.
In their own ways
they exemplify the change of consciousness
that will lead to a healthier, longer life for us all.

Part I

Living a Century

*F*ear less, hope more,

eat less, chew more,

whine less, breathe more,

talk less, say more,

hate less, love more,

and all good things will be yours.

— Swedish Proverb

The Ideal of Living Well

Besides being a great guy to talk to, Ben is a piece of evidence.
He is evidence of the truth "you are as you think."

It was just a business call. At least that's how Ben described it as we discussed book distribution. But when you're in my kind of "business" no call is ever *just* a call. They are always a bit more meaningful, metaphysically speaking.

Ben *happened* to call while I was writing the words you will soon read. This was his first time to call the School of Metaphysics. His business is selling what are called remainder books, in our case a print overrun surplus which resulted in a couple thousand books that needed a home. Ben's inquiry was an answer to my prayer. With three and possibly four books slated for publishing this year and limited warehouse space, we needed a compatible company that would buy and sell several of our older books. His call literally came out of the blue for he was responding to an intuitive message for help I had sent out some months ago.

Ben would modestly say he was doing his job. I would smile as I am privileged to see yet again the Universal Laws at work.

Then there's the "bit more" to Ben's call.

As we spoke I found Ben an engaging fellow. In the course of our ten minute conversation he spoke about life on the East coast of the U.S. and I about life in the Midwest. He told me he was a 70-year-old who had retired a while ago and come back to work because his wife said he was too cranky. He noted how he enjoyed his work and his life. He even shared a bit of philosophy telling me how he and his wife were on the Boardwalk and he noticed how obsessed we as Americans are with eating. "Everyone was eating," he said. "And I thought why don't you just smell the ocean air?" I commended him saying he reminded me of the people I was writing about in a book about health; people who live long, fulfilling lives.

Immediately, Ben responded. Turns out fourteen years ago Ben was in a car accident. "Doctors made a drugee out of me," he said. He needed two canes to walk and had no peripheral vision. One day he decided he was going to do strictly therapy. He was going off the dope. His doctors insisted he sign release forms so they wouldn't be liable, which he did. And now Ben swims three times a week, exercises every day, and drives.

He is a testimony to how the human spirit can cause health. And his testimony which I can now share with you is another expression of how those laws of the universe are constantly at work.

Before Ben and I parted company, I told him with his attitude and insight he'd probably live another 70 years. He said, "I'll be happy with another twenty, if I can continue to work and have some fun too."

Ben accepts his own mortality with grace and with humor. When he took control of his recovery, he also assumed control of his destiny. Now Ben is a man of ideals. Unlike those who immerse their minds in physical activity as a way to avoid contemplation of their own finiteness, he realizes the value of life's experiences. He knows he works because he has something valuable to contribute. He appreciates his good fortune, and it shows in his words and actions. He is free of fears about his mortality because he knows the connection between longevity and good health.

Most of us are like Ben. Too much of our lives are spent waiting until an experience happens before we ponder its significance. We work, we marry, we have children, we recreate. We settle into patterns of life – getting up at the same time of day, going to work, coming home, going to bed, only to awake and do it all over again. The degree to which this is true is the degree to which we await crisis. Crisis might come in the form of ending associations, such as divorce or being fired from your job, or it might arise through accident or injury, as it did for Ben. Crisis can present itself in the form of disease or the death of a relative or loved one. Each of these are terminations. They are the end of something. When an experience we have become accustomed to ends abruptly, seemingly without our pemission, we are forced to see the world differently. The loss of a house, the death of a parent, an adverse medical diagnosis, affect us in profound ways. At least we are forced to admit that we have lost someone or something; at most we question why and we discover life changing answers. No other experience shared by humanity seems to stimulate this more than facing our own finiteness. Coming to terms with mortality is a universal experience.

One of the most popular lecture topics offered by speakers in the School of Metaphysics over the last twenty years enables participants to deal with their own mortality in a meaningful way. As part of this presentation, audience members are asked to actively participate in a hypothetical situation provoking thought. The lecturer tells the audience s/he has been informed by their doctor that they only have one year to live. Once this idea is accepted, participants are asked to write down how they will spend this last year of life.

The speaker continues describing his topic for some time then tells the audience he has been informed that they do not have a year to live. By new test results they only have six months left on Earth. Again the audience is asked to record how they will spend the next 180 days.

After several more minutes of lecturing, the speaker informs the audience that a mistake was made, records were switched, and the correct analysis shows they are in exceptional health! These tests show the audience will live for years and years to come.

After giving time for this new information to be absorbed, the lecturer asks the audience how they will spend these future decades. Will they carry out their imagined plans from the hypothetical "death sentence" or will they continue to live just as they planned before this thought-generating exercise? The audience responses are always revealing and insightful.

After attending these lectures, most participants realize what they thought they were afraid of is in reality not what they fear at all. Most people can accept the idea that one day they will cease to live in the physical world. Most people have a system of beliefs that help them imagine existence beyond this life. Whether religious or even scientific, ideas of afterlife replace fear of the unknown. In most cases it is not death we fear, it is living.

By facing their own mortality, even if only through their imagination, the audience becomes a little more empowered to live a fuller, more rewarding life. They become more willing to share their thoughts and feelings with others. They are more adventurous, trying something new or fulfilling a long-held desire. Even without considering the spiritual roots of physical existence, such as religious concepts of afterlife or the possibility of reincarnation, most audience participants experience a renewed consciousness producing a more loving and purposeful existence. They come one step closer to knowing that physical life is a time to excel in learning thus enriching progression of the soul.

One of the most mind-expanding issues anyone faces is his own mortality. When you realize the fleeting nature of physical life, each moment becomes more precious to you. There is no time to waste so you become mindful of how you spend the time you have. The *quality* of your life becomes equally important.

Longevity may be a desire on everyone's list – "I want to live to see my grandkids have kids" – but increasingly as a society we are learning that what used to be true about longevity seems to be less and less the case. Individual strength, durability, resistance, resilience, health determines longevity for most of the world. Modern technology has supplanted many of the individual's natural resources that would, left uninterrupted, determine longevity. Yes, manmade insulin is a life saver, and extender, for thousands. And yes, manmade "lungs" can breathe for human lungs that gave up years ago.

Do we really want to live many years if you are unable to think and do and go as you desire? Our greatest fear is not dying but living with less than what we have come to expect and enjoy, living without what we value most. We are afraid that the freedom we enjoy in living will be lost; eyes that can see will suddenly be blind, legs that can move will suddenly be paralyzed, a mouth that can speak will be rendered mute, a brain that can record and access information will suddenly fail to perform on command. And so the quality of our life becomes perhaps even more important than the quantity.

The impact upon your consciousness of the brevity of physical life, whether it comes from your own desire for insight or from a doctor's warning of probable illness, can foster significant life changes. When made, these changes will extend the number of your healthy productive years. Internal physical changes in diet and exercise are commonplace. So are external physical changes, like moving to a different climate or out of the city for better air quality. These changes can aid merely by relieving the body of physical stress. But physical changes alone will not, cannot, ensure good health.

Neither his wife nor the retired Ben liked him very much. When you're cranky and restless, life loses some of its attractiveness. The luster also pales when you are critical, depressed, jealous, hateful, or generally unhappy and dissatisfied. The greatest changes we make in our lives are not the physical changes of what we eat, where we live, or even who we live with. The greatest transformations arrive in the form of new ideas about who we are, new motivations for caring for others, and new concepts of our reason for living. Longevity becomes desirable for those whose minds are filled with love, purpose, hope, ideals, and promise. When the consciousness is uplifted, the emotions and even the physical body follow suit, and this is according to those laws of the universe. The cause for health begins in the quality of the thinking. The life of the optimist, the positively progressive thinker and doer, is fulfilling no matter what the duration. And it is often of benefit to many others as well.

Such realizations are a way of life for those who have witnessed the coming and going of a century. Those who have lived that long are usually found in homes, not institutions. They are usually independent, not tied to machines that support their life. They are human encyclopedias of wisdom surpassing any computer program or television history show we'll ever create. Listening to the insightful experiences of those who have lived long, healthy lives is an education in the character, the attitudes, that favor longevity. The centenarians are those who have been where we want to go.

The typical scientific approach to learning from the centenarians is revealed in a university study of ninety-six centenarians in the southern United States. The objective was to determine why some people live more than 100 years. Searching for commonalties that would lead to greater longevity for us all, the scientists were surprised by what they discovered. They expected diet, lifestyle, and genetic make-up to be predominant factors for each of the participants. Yet the evidence did not support their preconceived hypotheses. In fact, these centenarians ranked highest in daily caloric intake which included large amounts of fat. They ate whatever they wanted! It was reported that the centenarian's ability to defy the rules of "good nutrition" mystifies scientists because they can't explain it.

What these scientists were encountering is the esoteric truth of longevity. These insights, well-known to metaphysicians, served to transcend scientific prejudices and open researchers' minds to the ruling power of creative thought. The study did reveal four commonalties in the centenarian's experiences.

The first is *optimism.* Anyone who accepts the power of thought knows a positive mental attitude causes all the things we value in life: good and lasting friendships, material and spiritual excellence, resilient health, and prosperity. One of the ladies interviewed counseled in this way, "Think positive! Don't waste time thinking negatively, do what you have to do." Researchers noticed a profound lack of depression among the centenarians, finding them "unbuggable" and not easily upset. The strong sense of optimism shared by these people was best described by a 105-year-old woman, "I know I'm coming close to the end, but I am glad to have been able to be here this long to see all this."

The second commonality for the centenarians was termed *engagement*. Engagement is the ability to commit to something of importance greater than yourself. This was illustrated by one man's deep religious faith. A churchgoer for more years than anyone else in his church, he never misses a service or meeting and no one makes a decision without his input. A woman described her faith as her constant motivation to be a better person. When asked why she thought she had lived over a hundred years, she said, "I figure the Lord's giving me more time to be a better person."

The third commonality is *activity* or *mobility*. Each of the centenarians engage in some form of physical activity daily. One man walks one mile from his home to the town square every day. A woman leads a group of youngsters in their eighties in mild aerobics. Another described how she was offered a new job serving as an historic home tour guide at age 97. Her first response was "Oh, I'm too old." Since the home was younger than she was, the reply was "You're a natural!" She's been serving as a tour guide in that home for over five years. By watching these centenarians you could easily tell they are not only physically active but mentally active as well, embracing discovery and newness in life continually.

The fourth commonality, and perhaps the most logically discerned, is *adaptability to loss*. All of the study participants had experienced the death of peers, many the death of siblings, and most the death of a spouse. The ability to continue in life, being flexible in the face of change, fosters an inner resolve to embrace the natural ebb and flow of existence. "It's wonderful to be alive now," one said. Another woman's 77-year-old daughter died peacefully of a heart attack the day before the centenarian was to be interviewed. She did not cancel her interview, saying it would be a tribute to her daughter. She shared memories of when her daughter was young. She recalled her daughter praying to God before becoming peaceful in sleep. The woman described her "loss" as giving back to God the gift he had given her.

In a time when one third of the population of the United States is over 55, it is well that we heed the wisdom of these elder citizens. The way they think and subsequently the way they live their lives can be an enlightening blessing for us all. No matter what our physical age, we can receive guidance and strength from the understanding born from experience. As we incorporate the four commonalties outlined in this study, we find the way to live a full and rewarding life which will, not incidentally, relieve any hesitations or fears of our own mortality. With optimism, engagement, activity, and adaptability, we can embrace life completely knowing the part we play in the scheme of creation. Whether our physical lifetime is only a decade or spans over a century, we will know we have lived well for our existence has served a purpose greater than ourselves.

Not long ago the United States Public Health Service reported that during a 76-year lifespan the average person can expect to have about 12 unhealthy years. This means most of us will experience 64 healthy years. This means in this country we will enjoy more healthy years than most individuals on the planet experience since the global average life span stands at 49 years of age.

We are truly blessed.

Imagine what will happen when governmental health organizations become curious about what *creates* health than what destroys it. We will all be more healthy. This is also true for allopathic (medical) professionals.

Consider this, a report from the *Journal of the American Medical Association* says those unhealthy years are spent coping with illnesses such as pneumonia, heart disease, cancer and diabetes, or with disabilities from work-related injuries or violence. If you think, as I do, that the quality of your thinking affects all aspects of your life including your health, then this report indicates that the average person is far more positively-oriented than pessimistic. There exists in most people in this country a healthy optimism to draw upon and, as we learned from those in their second century, optimism is the first key to longevity.

Optimism arises in a mind open to possibility. It is the result of a thinking individual whose imagination is acutely and purposefully active.

An optimist knows how to dream, and lives to make those dreams come true. An optimist expects the best, and holding ideals holy until they are a manifested reality. An optimist puts a smile on his face and yours, for optimism warms the heart while it allows the mind to soar. Optimism unites ideas and their makers. The synergy produced is remarkable.

Many experience synergy between spirit, mind, and body. The athlete calls it the burn or the high. The psychologist for years called it a peak experience, now it is known as quantum change. The devotee knows it as ectasy. Medical science calls it a miracle.

Miracles occur everyday. Falling in love. The birth of an eagerly anticipated child. Being at the right place at the right time with the right people. What you may not realize is that it is possible to *create* miracles in your life. Your potential for health and wholeness is unlimited. That potential is based on what you have within you, the state of your own consciousness. Understanding yourself as consciousness can be a challenge because the knowledge and practices that promote inner wisdom are not yet readily available. Yes, such knowledge exists throughout the world, particularly in the holy scriptures of each culture, but until this century instruction in consciousness has been offered only at secret schools such as the Vatican or in secret societies like the Freemasons to name two. What consciousness is, where it comes from and why it exists is not widely taught by parents or teachers to all of us. Although through the efforts of those who are committed to Enlightenment we can look forward to this changing in the coming decades.

Self consciousness distinguishes Mankind from all other life forms on this planet. Only man is capable of knowing himself as a creator. This makes him accountable while giving him dominion. In one of the most graphic examples, man, as creator, can unite human sperm and egg outside of the female womb to create a zygote but he has yet to give that potential human body a soul. It is well that we keep in mind man is practicing to *be like his Creator* but as yet he is not God. At this stage of our spiritual development, the most man can hope for is to bring his own soul to his creations. It has been said before that the greatest tragedy in life is to have the experience but miss the meaning. Consciousness is what enables us to ascertain and assess meaning, to make every experience fruitful.

How well you know yourself as the master of your life depends upon your willingness to respond to your potential. Master or slave, victor or victim, the reality lies not so much in our physical circumstances as in the way we choose to think of ourselves and others. It is universally true that a wise man will make a heaven from Hades while a fool will make a hell out of heaven. Our attitude about ourselves and our lives not only colors our experiences but indeed causes them to be what they are. The more you respect your capacity for mastery, the more you come to realize that the distance between health and illness is the distance between enlightenment and ignorance.

Understanding yourself as consciousness begins by realizing the separation between you, the thinking being, and the physical vehicle, your body. You probably own a car. You might own a Taurus, or maybe a Toyota. Your car might be a Chevrolet, a Mercedes or a Porsche. They are all a means of conveyance, a mechanical device that enables people to go from one place to another more quickly than by using only the body. Yet when you get into your car, your Ford, to go somewhere you don't become a Ford. You know that the Ford is a Ford. It is a car. It has its own composition and performs certain functions under your direction. When you get in that Ford there is no confusion in your mind as to who you are and what the Ford is.

Your physical body is just like your Ford. The physical body is a vehicle for the soul. It is a means of conveyance for consciousness to move from birth to death. The difficulty arises, and this is what promotes disease or illness, because we confuse who we are with this Ford that we are riding in. We begin to think that we are this Ford, and we forget to pay attention to who we are apart from this physical body. This becomes apparent in how people respond, or neglect to respond, to a common function of inner consciousness occuring every night – dreaming.

This is well illustrated in the words of actor Christopher Reeve, best known for his Superman roles, who was paralyzed in a 1995 fall from a horse. Even months after losing the vital connections that enable the legs to walk, hands to move, and even lungs to breathe, Reeves has said repeatedly that adjusting to the fact of his physical condition is a daily process. He talks of learning that he – the person who thinks and feels and desires – is separate from the body. Just because the body no longer responses to his wishes does not eliminate the wishes. Nor do the limitations of the body determine the person. Reeves speaks of dreaming. Like most people who experience physical impairment after birth, he is whole in his dream. Legs jump. Hands write. Torso turns. At will. Reeves says his challenge is realizing upon awakening that the body he once enjoyed, the body he still knows in his dreams, is no longer the body he has. It is a difficult way to learn a Universal Truth.

Those who do not understand the workings of subconscious mind and the nature of dreaming may think it cruel that the mind can allow us to believe something that is not true. The truth is we are not the bodies we inhabit. The soul is transcendent, existing before physical birth and after physical death. The soul is the real self, and dreaming is its means of communicating. Too few people take their dreams seriously. Most hurry through their day, carrying troubled concerns into sleep. The restless consciousness never knows stillness, thus peace eludes it; so does the rejuvenation sorely needed by an active mind. Dreaming is an experience that is beyond the waking, conscious state. It is the memory of experience in inner worlds. We may be living in a "Ford" in the outer, physical world, but in the inner world we may "drive" a Rolls Royce. In the inner levels of consciousness the blind can see, the lame can walk, the rich are poor, the average become outstanding.

Dreams are much more than wish-fulfillment or fantasies come true; that is the realm of daydreams not nocturnal ones. Our nighttime dreams are messages from the inner levels of our consciousness. They reflect the inner, subconscious mind's power to diagnose the state of our health – spiritually, mentally, emotionally and physically. Anyone desiring a sound mind and healthy body will draw upon this inner resource for instructive guidance and help in healing during times of need.

Interpreting dreams is a skill, like reading or communicating, that is taught and learned. By learning the Universal Language of Mind, the language used during dreams, everyone can understand the meaning of these inner experiences. Soon the language becomes the means for a two-way communication which strengthens the power of both the conscious part and the subconscious part of your consciousness. In time you learn to exist with ease in the inner worlds becoming aware of the point of origin of your physical existence. Intuitive development is quickened and soul progression is accelerated.

The nature of all life is to grow. Whether the simplest of life forms or the most complex, the urge for growth is constantly present. The desire of the spirit is for wholeness, completeness, maturity. Your innate urge is toward growth which in itself is the state of being called wellness. That urge can be described as a willingness to sacrifice your energy to something higher than yourself. Be it a mother giving all her energy to her children, a statesman giving all his energy to his country, or a monk giving all his energy to God, sacrifice is the ability to transcend personal ego for the good of All. This is engagement in its highest manifestation.

When you seek the fulfillment of that inner spiritual urge, working in alignment with the laws of the universe, ever-deepening awareness is yours. Your mind is positively directed toward what you love and your energy is boundless. Your health – spiritually, mentally, emotionally, and physically – is exceptional. But resist growth, try to keep conditions and even yourself from changing, and you find deterioration. Your spirit weakens; your belief in yourself wanes. Your mind tires as reserves of energy are consumed by the conflicts without being replenished by the insight of resolve. Your emotions become centered around the limits you have set until they erupt because they can no longer be contained. Your body is the final battlefield, where invaders whether viral or bacterial find the weakened immune system and malnourished cells fertile ground for conquering. Resist growth and you invite illness to enter your life.

It is a universal truth that the nature of the mind is motion. Therefore it requires an act of intelligence and will to direct that motion toward productive ends. This is why setting goals works for those desiring to achieve. It is why creating positive images of what you desire quickens the attainment of them. Intelligence and will is why people born of the same race, sex, economic class, cultural traditions, and even in the same family can be so very different, one a success the other a failure, one charismatic the other a misanthrope, one healthy the other sick all his life. Remember the centenarian's third key is activity, and the motion that extends life is much more than just muscle-bumping. It is the movement of energy, of chi or ki or prana, from the inner levels of existence to the outer. It is the vital life force that feeds your physical body enabling it to live.

The physical world is the final expression of mind. The physical manifestation of the mind's motion is most readily identified as change. In fact, for this reason the nature of the physical is change. One of the great benefits of five hundred years of science is the recent technology enabling us to see the molecular structure of the chair you are setting on, or the clothes you are wearing or the physical body, the "Ford", you are riding in. From our removed viewpoint, we know the chair, clothes, and our bodies as solid. Magnify these and we find particles of energy dancing in intricate formations. Even though your body seems firm and hard, it is constantly in motion. It is constantly changing. The oxygen-laden air you inspire is not the same air you exhale. It has undergone chemical changes while inside your body therefore you expire carbon dioxide as a waste product you no longer need.

The beauty of the universe is that everything is useable. What is a waste product for man, and toxic to his well-being, is necessary for the existence of other life forms, plantlife. The waste of plants – oxygen – becomes the nourishment needed for man to live. Changes in the universe, when in cooperation with Universal Law, allow for growth. When man obstructs natural change dis-ease results. Whether the waste products of chemicals intended to relieve suffering or the waste products of a nation that man has failed to find a use for, to recycle, these by-products remain until man finds a use for them. Often, until then, they are the source of more problems.

The centenarian's adaptability rises from being connected with the universe. It is at once a surrender to forces greater than themselves and a conquering of their own attachments to that which is temporary. This sense that nothing is ever completely destroyed, only changed in form, frees us to embrace creation with gratitude and with hope.

Healing is the ability for man to create wholeness. Where there is healing there is no waste, only the complete expression of energy. Thus when someone speaks of "healing a nation", they are expressing a desire for unity born from cooperation, where all parts work together to create a larger whole, and all intelligences share a purpose of the common good. Where this is present a human being can exist as a viable healthy entity, and so can a planet.

Most people react to their bodies.

The body says it is hungry, so its owner feeds it. The body says it is too warm, so its owner sheds clothing or takes a cold shower. The body says it cannot go on without rest, so its owner sleeps. Simple and universal needs.

But what about the person with arthritis who says, "I can't get around like I used to." The person with stomach complaints who says, "I just can't eat spicy food anymore." Or the person who has endured a heart attack saying, "I have to slow down, I guess I'll decline that promotion and raise." Or someone with skin cancer who believes, "I can't go out in the sun anymore." Based upon currently accepted thinking, these statements seem reasonable. But there is no denying the loss of mobility, freedom, fulfillment, or enjoyment that these statements describe. And there is a drain upon mental energies when illness strikes. There are also emotional debts to pay.

Here one of the most profound and enduring questions asked by man applies: which came first, the chicken or the egg? With our list of unfortunate sufferers, which came first, the physical symptoms of disease or dis-ordered thoughts? As you learn about our research, particularly in the health analyses, I hope you will be able to answer this question with deeper insight, for according to the universal principles which govern creation there is indeed an answer which applies to anyone, anywhere, any time.

When the truth is known how we think about our bodies often provides a clue as to why they are functioning, or malfunctioning, as they are. There is no doubt in the mind of anyone who has suffered from arthritis that the pain associated with the movement of affected joints restricts movement. Simple acts, opening a can, combing your hair, or rising from a chair, can seem unbearable. The physical reality of the body's limitations affect the mind. The mind must adjust its attitude to those physical limitations – "I can't get around like I used to" – unless it becomes more self aware. Part of that awareness is realizing the universal truth, thought is cause. The advantage of knowing that thought is cause is not avoiding or ignoring the physical body as some might be tempted to believe. The advantage is appreciating the body that much more. For with knowledge comes power: the power to be attentive, to identify and respond to needs, to create attitudes conducive to good, sound health.

Being educated in the simple facts of how the human body functions is like learning the basic workings of a car. Just as it is helpful to know the signs that a wheel alignment is needed for your car, so it is helpful to realize when your body might need a spinal adjustment because your skeletal system is misaligned. In both cases, early detection and response will give you peace of mind and can save you time and money.

Knowing how to *respond* to what your body is telling you ensures well-being. The more aware we are of what causes our bodies to perform as they do the easier it is to guarantee good health. With so many over-the-counter drugs, it is far too easy to ignore what your body is telling you. The body says it is nauseous, so its owner takes a chemical to alter the body chemistry masking the symptom. Most people believe they are responding when they take a drug, prescribed or otherwise. They believe relief from pain is an equivalent to a cure. Unfortunately it is not. Read the warnings and list of side effects that must accompany every prescription. You will quickly see one of the effects the chemical produces is immediate symptomatic relief of what ails you *and* it will also cause repercussions in other parts of the body. The body is a whole system, and drugs affect the whole system. This tendency to deny wholeness is the first failure to respond and it is the first step toward illness.

A colleague of mine spent all his adult years in the business of filling prescriptions for those in need. In his retirement years he found the time to pursue his interests, one of which was studying applied metaphysics. His experience brings a unique perspective to how our society has become divided; on one hand dependent on the instant relief from pain that drugs bring, on the other hand abhorring the pain and destruction of lives that illegal drugs bring. In both cases the problem isn't the chemicals, sometimes they are needed. The problem is in ourselves, an unwillingness to look at ourselves honestly and be responsible for what we see.

"As a pharmacist I was in practice from 1941 to 1990. During the first years of our pharmacy we filled about 20 prescriptions a day. There were very few tranquilizers or other mind-altering drugs on the market during the first 10 years. By 1990, when I retired, there were hundreds of tranquilizers available and they were badly abused. We filled up to 200 prescriptions a day.

"I have always been concerned with the question, 'What is the cause of the illness?' Covering up the symptoms does not get to the cause that is necessary for a cure. I would often say, 'He is not long for this world!' when someone who had lost their purpose in life would come to have a prescription filled. This was especially true of retired folks. I became more and more disturbed as I realized that few people really wanted to hear that their illness might be related to their negative thoughts and attitudes. I often asked the question: 'Do you really want a tranquilizer?' Some patients were interested and wanted to know more, but most considered their situation as 'fate.'

"I see the Intuitive Health Analyses as a service to anyone who wants to maintain good health. These intuitive reports relate the mental, emotional and physical disorders and give the thoughts and attitudes causing the problems. Guidance is given to help the individual make any attitudinal changes necessary. Once the person has insight into the cause of their problem they have a choice of the direction they wish to take to improve their future health. Contrast this to the fear that is often instilled in a patient who hears, 'you must take this drug!' Perhaps the following month that same drug may be proven to have serious side effects or is declared worthless.

"The public needs to be educated on health matters. I do see this coming as more and more health articles are being published in the nation's major magazines and newspapers pointing out the relationship between mind and body."

Sometimes those requesting an Intuitive Health Analysis who are taking drugs for a medically diagnosed condition will ask if they should be taking the chemical, if there are harmful side effects. The analysis does not prescribe, rather it *de*scribes the chemical interactions occurring in the body. When addressing the introduction of manmade drugs, analyses tend to merely comment upon whether they are beneficial or detrimental to the body, whether they are producing the expected effect. This is particularly important when the drugs are forcing interactions that would otherwise not arise. These forced interactions are typically called "side effects" and the list of possible complications or even damage to the body accompanies every drug marketed in the U.S. Few people take time to read them, and many mix medicines at their own peril. Health analyses do not interfere with conventional medical diagnosis although they can upon occasion recommend seeking it.

The analysis will report the complications arising from a major disorder, many times informing the person of drug side effects that he might not have learned about any other way. Thus a man discovers that his daily intake of broccoli, meant as an antioxidant to ward off aging and cancer, is reducing the effectiveness of a physician-prescribed blood thinner. The vitamin K found in broccoli and other green leafy vegetables helps the blood clot which in this case was neutralizing the intended benefit of the drug. A woman learns that the salt substitute she is using to control high blood pressure is elevating the level of potassium in her body and causing even more pressure to be put upon her heart. Recommendations for herbs that will help balance her bodily system and enhance the flavor of her food are given. Most doctors are nutritionally ignorant, they didn't learn about it in school and they don't have time to learn about it now. They just don't know all the chemical interactions that occur in the body and probably very few people if any have memorized all the known knowledge. An Intuitive Health Analysis is much more likely to identify and address these interactions because it draws upon subconscious knowledge, going beyond conscious memory and reasoning, perceiving the individual as a whole organism.

When examining how the body exchanges energies from natural sources, intuitive analysis is unparalleled. Because these readings report the condition of your body right now, they give amazing insight into where imbalances are occurring and what can be done to remedy them. Personal assessment and personal recommendations for optimal health. Thus a person wanting to know if fruit juices, particularly prune, will alleviate a tendency toward constipation learns that buttermilk is a better choice because the buttermilk will supply the natural intestinal bacteria needed for elimination while being easier on a stomach prone to ulcers. Another discovers a supplementary vitamin is not being absorbed by the body because of how and when the person is consuming it. A new mother learns that her fussy newborn is reacting to the caffeine level in the mother's milk which can easily be remedied. Once informed, the individual must respond. When you learn what to do and how to do it, you are the one in charge of your health. This is the great challenge knowledge brings. There are no magic pills in any form, just a series of adjustments in attitude and action that will enable mind and body to exist in active peace.

Chemical changes are not a replacement for changes in the heart and mind. Those who are not so much concerned with healing as they are with ending the awareness of pain find this idea difficult to accept. So does the drug addict and the alcoholic. Drugs are without question abused in our society. As a result we find other forms of abuse prevalent as well. When individuals do not look for the cause of their pain, only ways to hide it, whatever is promoting the pain escalates until it manifests in a fit of rage against a loved one or neighbor, or in a raging disease in the body. When healing is desired there is no place for denial, there is only room for admittance and repentance.

By educating ourselves and our children to the unlimited possibilities of the human mind, we can learn the kinds of thoughts and actions that heal. Time and again, health analyses describe the astounding power of the mind. And repeatedly they indicate that whether the mind's power heals or slays, creates or destroys, *depends upon the desire to learn and the willingness to be changed by what is learned.*

Taking charge of your health requires self-examination.

It does not have to be mentally or emotionally painful, although it can be. We must learn that pain, wherever it is experienced, exists to draw the attention to something that is wrong. A sprained ankle causes sufficient pain that we favor that leg, giving the injured one the time and space to heal. Without the pain we would continue to place weight on the bruised tissues causing further and eventually irreparable damage. Pain then promotes the change needed for healing to take place. Masking the capacity for the consciousness to be warned is paving the way for future problems.

Mental or emotional pain also draws the attention to what is wrong, only instead of a disorder in the body this dis-ease exists in our attitudes. The emotional pain of divorce can come from broken promises or fears of loneliness or deceits confessed or shattered pride. Fail to realize the reason the pain exists and you set your destiny to repeat the patterns of thinking, mistakes, that culminated in the present dilemma. The cure is never found by escaping into alcohol, drugs, or therapy. Nor does it come from terminating the situation where the pain arises. Admitting your weaknesses alone is not enough. There must be a change of mind, a change of heart, for healing to occur. Whatever is causing you pain, the cure is found in self-revelation that transforms.

Intuitive Health Analyses promote self-realization. They empower people to make transformations that heal mind and body. Information received in this kind of analysis does not come from examining the physical body alone, in fact, the body does not even have to be within the intuitive reporter's presence. From the inner levels of consciousness patterns of thinking, harmonious or inharmonious, productive or destructive, are seen and their effects upon the body can be traced. Intuitive diagnosis of the individual's state of health is derived from the direct grasp of truth available in the inner levels of consciousness. Those who provide the analysis have prepared for this work by years of concentration and meditation practices.

Health analyses give new meaning to early detection. By intuitively examining the way energy is being used, many times trouble areas become apparent *before* physical disorders arise. As you will soon learn, Intuitive Health Analyses were never designed to replace any form of treatment currently available. From surgery to acupuncture, from psychiatry to prayer, the health analyses recommend those treatments which accelerate recovery and restore wholeness.

As we progress into the next stage of Mankind's development, the stage beyond twentieth century technology, the Intuitive Health Analysis will increasingly become the "first opinion" secured for our health and well-being.

The Need to Know the Truth

Preventive mastectomies.

The idea has been around for several years spurred by genetic research which isolated genes that may indicate a propensity for breast and ovarian cancer. The idea is if the gene runs in your family and you have it, then should the potential offending body part be removed the potential cancer cannot grow where the fertile tissue is no longer present.

Researchers call it a gamble. The medical predictions are that a high-risk, 30-year-old woman who has her breasts removed can gain from three to five years of life. Those having ovaries removed can gain a few months to a few years of life. The trouble is not all seemingly cancer-prone women will actually get cancer. Science has yet to learn what the determining factor is. When asked, the lead researcher at the Dana Farber Cancer Institute in Boston was quoted as saying, "We don't have a crystal ball."

Maybe that's the real point. Maybe it's time for medical science to rethink the theories which have guided its practices and shaped its conclusions. Maybe it's time for researchers and physicians to expand their view of the species they seek to aid.

Intuitive Health Analyses report what is present and what is forming in the consciousness of the person receiving the reading. This gives new meaning to the term "early detection". These reports are secured from the inner levels of consciousness. They are metaphysical evidence of dis-ease. This means the inner subconscious mind is used to perceive disorders at their point of origin. And that point of origin is how we think.

This idea is simple. So simple, it is rejected by the new but well-established physicians found in most hospitals and clinics today. I say new because it is only in this century that medical associations and networks have proliferated and successfully ostracized, through legislation and publicity, health care that has stood the test of time. These methods seek to heal without technology, methods like midwifery, acupuncture, naturopathy. Each of these affirm and rely upon the individual's responsibility and power for resilience and recovery.

The concept is fundamental. The quality of our thinking, how we view ourselves and our world, is what determines the quality of our outer life as well as the inner environment. Generally speaking, an optimistic, enthusiastic outlook upon life gives you the impulse to joyfully, and fitfully, arise to meet the new day. Anticipatory thoughts stimulate the body to prepare; hormones flow, breathing deepens, digestion moves, circulation increases, all systems are go. A pessimistic, forlorn outlook on life breeds self-doubt and a host of real or imagined fears signaling the body to swing from one extreme to another. Here we find the seeds for hypoglycemia and diabetes, for high and low blood pressure, for irregularities in the alimentary system or in the menstrual cycle.

The quality of our thinking determines both inner and outer harmony, inner and outer productivity, inner and outer health. The concept is as simple as the colloquialisms in our daily language: he's a pain in the neck, the loss broke my heart, the news turned my stomach, he vented his spleen. Each are metaphors describing how a thought or emotion is connected to a specific body part. These are the connections being detailed by SOM research, and revealed daily through intuitive analysis.

The truth is conventional medical research supports what Intuitive Health Analyses reveal. The reason medical researchers are not farther along is the tendency to see the human body as an end, in and of itself. There is little consideration of the soul or spirit which animates that body, providing it with the life force necessary to it to move, talk, walk, and think. This is a huge oversight that keeps leading researchers to more questions rather than answers to existing ones.

In the case of the breast cancer gene, as the medical research increases so does the confusion. The original idea was that discovering a breast cancer gene would lead not only to a test but to simple ways to prevent the disease from arising. That has not been the case because not everyone who suffers from the disease has the defective genes. The cancer can run in families but it doesn't always, and the big question remains unanswered, "Why?"

Oddly enough the medical establishment would probably be closer to the answer if you knew the name Bechamp as well as Pasteur. Antoine Bechamp and Louis Pasteur, both 1800's French microbiologists, set the stage for what we know as modern medicine. They engaged in a scientific and philosophical debate concerning the cause of disease. The fact that Bechamp lost the contest is the reason why current medical research and knowledge is not more advanced than it is.

Pasteur concluded that disease is solely caused by germs. Bacteria (or microbes) invade the body from the outside causing damage, disease, and death. He promoted this theory of disease, called monomorphism. Monomorphism means a microorganism is static and unchangeable. It is what it is. Bechamp promoted pleomophism meaning that microorganisms change. They go through stages of development evolving into various forms within their life cycle. From this Bechamp believed that sometimes the germs might be disease-causing and at other times not. Pasteur's work led to the present-day medical model of drugs that kill the germs.

That model is quickly breaking down. Antibiotics are a perfect example. Drugs that sweep through the human body killing every living organism, including friendly bacteria your body relies upon for proper function, are failing to accomplish their mission. It seems the germs mutate, just as Bechamp suspected. As is true with any life form, germs change in order to survive. The chemicals that killed them yesterday no longer work today. A recent, and most alarming, illustration of a germ's fight for life is Stapholoccocus, the infection common in every hospital. "Staph" no longer responds to the antibiotic designed to kill it.

Since germs are always finding a home in the human body, it is Bechamp's work, not Pasteur's, that will further research so we can learn how to cure physical disease. Modern medicine must change. Research needs to center upon discovering what stimulates germs to change, to move from benign to deadly. This answer may very well lie in the work of another Bechamp-Pasteur contemporary – Claude Bernard.

Bernard believed it was actually the environment or milieu that is all important to the disease process. How a microbe changes and evolves is a result of the environment to which it is exposed. Germs change *according to* the environment to which they are exposed therefore disease originates from within the body and how it develops or manifests is a function of the internal terrain. Bernard's theory will probably draw us closer to the truth; certainly SOM research supports it.

What happened? Disease is not new. Why aren't we farther along in knowing the cause and cure for what impairs and eventually kills us?

As has been the case so many times, the more vocal, willful, well-connected and money-backed individual prevailed thereby setting the course of history. In this case it was Pasteur. His ideas have indeed dominated the scientific community a century beyond his own lifetime. They were easy to buy and sell because they meant man is a victim of his environment, the germ has all the power and the best you can ever do is stay as germ-free as possible. Certainly sanitation plays a large part in creating a healthy outer environment but it does not cure all manners of disease. The eternal problem with this theory is illustrated in the question, "If germs are the cause of disease then why didn't I get sick when everyone else at the office came down with the flu?" Ironically, Pasteur, as he lay on his deathbed, indirectly acknowledged Bechamp's work by saying, "Bernard was correct, the microbe is nothing, the terrain is everything."

Pasteur's theory prevailed however and as a result, at least in the Western world, the state-of-the-art treatment of disease is allopathic (drug-based) medicine. When a body is out of balance, physicians attempt to reestablish equilibrium first through drugs, then through surgery. The general effect is the removal of symptoms instead of elimination of the ultimate cause of the ailment. Drugs do not stop the pain of disease, they merely interrupt your body's faculty for alerting your brain that something is wrong. Something is still wrong. Drugs then become a way of denying what that something is.

The 20th century theory says most disease is caused by germs, or some form of static disease-causing microbe. In order to get well you kill the germs. *Kill* the microbes. *Kill* whatever is making you sick. Thus we have drugs and antibiotics. We also have a host of treatments that kill not only the offenders but the host as well. We have poison (chemotherapy), burning (radiation), and slashing (surgery) as acceptable and even desirable methods of disease control. These are not used as a last resort. They are a daily means of health care throughout the United States and abroad.

For most people in the West the allopathic nature of health care fosters a false sense of security, a weakness of human resolve, and a capricious extension on a progressively deteriorating quality of life. Even in cases where drugs can kill an offending organism or surgery remove it, if the factors which produced the climate for dis-order – Bernard's milieu – continue to exist then the problem will recur. It does, and it will until we become more invested in finding cause and cure within ourselves rather than looking for a place to put blame and someone who can provide a quick fix. Even with, and maybe because of, its widespread societal acceptance and omnipresent availability, modern medicine is in its twilight years. The medicine of science and technology has existed long enough for us to determine what in reality are breakthroughs and what are breakdowns.

Hopefully the 21st century model of health care will be very different from what has come before. Hopefully the desire for more personal control of health will shape this concept. I predict that the acceptable model by the year 2100 will find its foundation in a concept forsaken in the 1800's, although its roots will span seven continents and extend back through millinnia. The new model will be based upon the theory that most disease is caused by an imbalance in the body brought about by *internal disruptions*.

Initially these will be viewed as physical imbalances: nutritional, electrical, structural, toxicological, or biological. Balance is reestablished in the body by working with it, not against it. Cooperating with the body means the kinds and quality of foods eaten will become more important than speed and convenience. Acupuncture will assume the place of respectability in Western science that it has held for over 2500 years in China as a natural means to regulate all systems of the body by stimulating the chromosomal meridians. Chiropractic care, which has survived repeated attempts by organized allopathic practitioners to force it into exile, will ensure a sound body structure enabling full sensory communication and conducive to muscular movement. Homeopathy will replace drugs used to offset toxicity in our world and our lives.

This 21st century model will be a synthesis of the best health care known to mankind. It will combine systems of healing into truly wholistic care. From traditional Chinese medicine to homeopathy, from AyurVeda of India to Greek medicine, each will offer their wisdom to aid man to be whole. Hippocrates, the father of modern medicine, said that although health is the natural state of humans, disease is also a natural process that follows an organic pattern. During an illness there are specific times when a physician can intercede, assisting his patient in restoring health. Hippocrates called these times "opportune moments", moments when balance can be restored. Any knowledge that can help the physician to recognize these moments is worthy not only of attention but of respectful employment.

When a physician has the knowledge and freedom to draw upon the wisdom of the world to heal his patient we will see a revolution in health care move across the face of the globe.

Idealistic? Yes. Possible? Yes, in fact inevitable. Evidence of this model is already apparent in the lives of health-minded people. These men and women take greater care in where they live and how they live. Even your doctor will encourage a change in the food you eat, increased physical exercise, cleaner air and less stress. The more we seek to eat nourishing foods, stimulate the body through movement, embrace healthy atmospheres and lifestyles while abandoning health-threatening ones, the more we realize these actions alone do not ensure long-lasting health. Everyone knows someone who has always done the right thing and she was diagnosed with ulcers or he died of a heart attack at a young age. What is the determining factor? Why does one twin manifest a health problem while the other does not? Their genetic makeup is as close as you will find and they are raised with similar environments. The answer lies in what determines "internal disruptions". What causes a single gene to go awry, manifesting cancer and becoming an internal assassin? In the end the only answer that makes sense is the owner of the body, the individual himself. This is a concept the systems of healing respect. From Chinese medicine's understanding that health begins with an understanding of nature and the laws that govern it to the naturopath's premise that every living cell in an organized body is endowed with an instinct of self-preservation which is sustained by an inherent vital life force, each honors the individual's capacity for healing.

Voltaire once said, "The art of medicine consists of amusing the patient while nature cures the disease."

Based upon his other writings, Voltaire knew that laughter is the best medicine because it causes the mind to embrace perspective while releasing trouble. The state of internal environment is paramount to health, and that state is ruled by you, the thinking being, the intelligence that makes you who you are, the spirit that gives you life. When the mind is at peace, the body is calm, following suit. When the mind is in turmoil, the body fights itself. The first internal environment is your attitude, this then determines the internal environment of your body.

For several years now the conventional Western medical establishment has discussed the impact of mental and emotional stress upon health. For some, I believe this is their effort to move toward becoming healers. They encourage patients to fight and defeat cancer by imaging good cells gobbling the bad cells. They recommend meditation for their highly stressed patients, particularly those prone to heart disease and heart failure. These physicians pair the best that modern technology has to offer with ways the dis-eased person can help themselves. He or she is the kind of physician we all hope we have should the need for medical help arise in our own lives.

Most people who choose medical science as a career want to be of service, they want to heal people. They are idealistic and altruistic. In time the reality of medical practice moves them away from the hope of curing and into what can chemically or surgically be done to save lives, or prolong them. For some, practicing medicine leads them to different conclusions. These physicians believe that killing a germ is not a prescription for health. They have seen too many medically treated people live less than fulfilling lives in bodies weakened by the therapies that were intended to help. They have seen some people restored to health without treatment while others receiving treatment falter, and they want to know why. These physicians realize modern medicine must move beyond Pasteur's legacy and begin to consider something other than a germ as the cause of man's disease and suffering.

The idea that the way you think influences the health or illness of your body is not new. It is ancient knowledge – far beyond the state-of-the-art discoveries of modern man – firmly rooted in what is natural to man, animal, plant, to all of creation. Hippocrates, the father of modern medicine, respected this wisdom: "The natural healing force within each of us is the greatest force in getting well." It is ironically comical to muse what he might think of what has become of his ideas. I'm sure he must be delighted to see the recent changes in the consciousness of those who want to serve. Natural healing is a concept whose time has come for us here in the technologically-centered Western world. And the first step toward natural healing is to accept the individual's power to determine his or her well-being and longevity.

Consider this list of ten pointers for a long and healthy life published in *Parade Magazine* (March 20, 1994):

1] Cherish your choices and maintain control of your own life.

2] Commit yourself to your passions in work and love—and embrace the conflicts and juggling involved.

3] Do more than one thing well.

4] Stop being afraid of real intimacy.

5] Risk being yourself, who you really are.

6] Pay attention to what's going on, the changes in your body and the outside world, the feelings of those you love and those with whom you work.

7] Risk new things, risk new ways, risk failing, risk mistakes, risk pain.

8] Use technologies and medical advances if they enhance or sustain your life—but beware of those that take choice away from you.

9] Be a part of the changing community.

10] Live it all.

Every pointer requires the individual to participate in a particular kind of thinking. Like your mother always told you, "It's the thought that counts." She was right.

The body is meant to function perfectly, indeed never aging or wearing out. Transplants have taught us that. Fifty-year-old kidneys function for another fifty or more when placed in an eighteen-year-old body. The human body functions according to Universal Law unless interrupted. Should it occur, the interruption comes in the form of thoughts and attitudes which bring the susceptibility for disease into the body. The need to know how attitude directly affects physical health is, in most cases, more important than diagnosis of the physical condition because just as attitude sets the stage for physical dis-ease it also governs the rate and duration of health recovery. Every physician can tell you stories about the amazing will to live that their patients have exhibited. To be healthy throughout our lives we must not wait until pain, disability, and disease come to draw upon inner resources. We must value attitude daily.

The need to know the truth was the impetus for developing the Intuitive Health Analyses.

Humanity must learn how attitudes are constructed so we are free to be as healthy as we desire. We must be self-reflective. If we are to take charge of our health we must reinforce healthy attitudes in ourselves and change the diseased ones. Learning what those attitudes are and how best to use them for health has been a large part of School of Metaphysics research for over a quarter of a century. Discovering how the findings apply to you personally is the best reason to seek intuitive guidance.

Intuition is the direct grasp of truth. Intuition operates beyond the everyday thoughts produced by the outer, physical mind. Clearly perceiving beyond the millions of pieces of information in the brain, the inner mind, disciplined and refined, exhibits astounding insight. Of its many faculties – which range from clairvoyance to out-of-body experience or astral travel, from telekinesis to knowledge of existence before physical birth and after physical death – the capacity to identify points of origin is by far the most useful for health and longevity. What arises from this ability to discern cause is unparalleled in any of man's other sciences.

By reporting the thoughts and attitudes existing in the mind, the lines of probability can be traced to their manifestation in the physical body, foretelling of potential areas of imbalance that will lead to disease. This is what occurs during an Intuitive Health Analysis. Most scientific studies examine the physical manifestations and workings of disease. Intuitive Health Analyses examine the energy disruptions and blockages in the mind and follow them as they express into the body as disease.

Scientific studies that seek to understand the effects of stress in our lives verify this intimate connection between mind and body. There is no longer any question that a person's mental and/or emotional condition directly affects the functioning of his body. One study finds people under continuous personal or work stress for more than a month were shown to be 2 1/2 times more susceptible to colds than other people. Another shows that chronic stress unleashes hormones and other chemicals that suppress the body's immunity, its ability to successfully fight invaders that cause disease. Still another concludes that people can have the same things going on in their lives – such as medical school exams – but have very different levels of stress and immune suppression. As an expert on stress and immunity at the National Institute of Health in Bethesda, Maryland, put it, "Stress is not what happens to you, it's how you respond to it." By learning more about stress responses, the hope is that new ways to help people avoid illness will be found.

An Intuitive Health Analysis gives you this kind of education. It paints a clear picture of the way you see your world. How you view yourself, your loved ones, your coworkers, even the stranger who took your place in line, becomes apparent as your dominant attitudes are described. Undesirable characteristics produce the discord in our lives and, if left to flourish, eventually promote dis-ease in the body. From arrogance to self-pity, from carelessness to blame, from cowardice to stubbornness, "stress" takes on a new meaning when it is elucidated. When something is going wrong, causing health problems, intuitive analysis goes beyond pinpointing the cause, it tells you what you can do to correct the problem. The reports do not mince words. They are at times direct and bluntly honest, at other times almost poetic; the analysis tends to reflect the person receiving it. Regardless of delivery, every Intuitive Health Analysis describes how the individual's learning is affecting him on a soul level. This reason alone makes this analysis a perfect place to begin for anyone who wants to be in charge of his or her health.

Intuitive Health Analyses exist as a way for people to be healthy and whole. Dr. Daniel Condron, Chancellor of the College of Metaphysics and author of **Permanent Healing**, likes to say that when you are severely ill is not the best time to seek the type of health analysis we offer. "Although intuitive reports have enlightened people, when they turn to us as a last resort that is not the time to get a health analysis because the report is not diagnostic. Intuitive information descibes your health condition - mentally, emotionally and physically - at the time it is given."

A conductor of intuitive consultations for two decades, Dr. Condron calls the analysis the best preventive measure available for staying healthy. "The phenomenal research conducted by the School of Metaphysics has spared many people unnecessary heartache and it has in many cases saved them a lot of money." It has also answered parents' questions concerning their children, helped sons and daughters accept a parent's impending death, helped others to place problems in perspective while empowering some to make significant changes in their inner lives. These analyses probe beyond what is immediately apparent, accessing depths beyond the realm of psychological or religious counseling. From the karmic implications of disease to impaired genetic mind patterns, our research is unveiling the complete nature of health and disease. In the process we are learning a great deal about healing.

We are much more than flesh and bones.
    Our bodies seem finite, solid. But they are in reality compositions of molecules, atoms, and subatomic particles constantly in motion. Energy held together by the magnetic force of thoughts, be they memories from the past or imagined hopes of the future, be they personal or professional, spiritual or secular. Our thoughts and emotions about what happens in our lives determines whether we are mentally adept or incompetent, emotionally comfortable or awkward, physically whole or infirmed. It is not so much the amount of energy we have as it is how we use that available energy that makes life worth living. The intelligence, that unique spark in every living person, is what makes all the difference. After all, when reduced down to its components of water, calcium, gold, and other elements, the physical human body looks nothing like a person and costs under ten dollars.
    I have always been amazed that all human bodies are basically the same, made of the same materials in similar pattern, yet they are so very different in size, shape, texture, and yes, health. Intuitive research explains why. Each analysis describes the way energy is being used or, in the case of disease, abused. The thoughts that misuse the mind's energy produce imbalance first in the mind then in the emotions and finally in the physical body. Once identified for what they are, these harmful or deficient attitudes can be eliminated by replacing them with beneficial and fertile ways of thinking. This efficient use of mental energy produces harmony between the mind and emotions and balance within the body.
    The best available treatment to restore balance – whether it comes from Chinese medicine, Ayurveda of India, Greek medicine, homeopathy, or modern medicine of Western science – is complemented by the Intuitive Health Analysis. The former restores balance in the ailing body which aids the mind toward clarity and the emotions toward equanimity. Both

absolutely necessary for health to be restored. The latter empowers the individual to transform his consciousness which is necessary for healing to occur. When you are healed, the way you use energy has changed leaving no avenue for the old disorder to recur.

Healing frees the spirit to soar so you can live life completely, accomplishing your dreams and fulfilling your soul's purpose. This is the future of mankind. A world where increasing numbers of people are intuitively aware of their destiny and able to enact it through the power of reasoning. Whole. Complete. Healthy.

Increasingly, Intuitive Health Analyses will become a widely accepted, integral part of individualized wholistic health care in the 21st century.

Intuitive Analysis
The Coming Revolution in Health Care

When I was seventeen years old, I had what every teenager dreams of – living quarters separate from their parents.

Actually, I lived only a hundred yards away from their small one bedroom house, but the one gigantic room above the family business made for a great attic apartment for me. One Friday evening a few friends and I returned from a movie to share opinions and secrets until our curfew alarm sounded. At one point, the discussion became particularly engrossing, and I found myself seeing what looked like a light surrounding my friend's head. It was as if he glowed. I wouldn't call it a halo, after all the discussion was not particularly holy, but there was this emanation of what seemed to be light.

This was not the first time I had seen the light. I can remember this phenomenon occurring while talking with people. But for some reason this night I decided to pursue it further.

"It must be the lighting in the room," I thought. This was my first hypothesis to prove or disprove. There must be a simple physical explanation. To this point in my life I had sought to make sense of life by seeking logical, physically-rooted reasons for my experiences. This arose from a foundation of loyal belief in the purposefulness of everything. I thoroughly believed no sane person every does anything without a reason, and that everything has a reason for being, even when I don't know what it is or when upon finding out do not like what I discover. So I got up and turned on a floor lamp. And then a hall light. The artificial light did not make the light I was seeing go away.

My next idea was perhaps I saw the light because of where I was sitting in relationship to the person talking. So I moved to another chair. Then I tried the floor. I found it didn't matter where I moved in the room. It might not happen right away but pretty soon I would begin to see this light again.

My next thought began to bridge the gap between a physical reason and a nonphysical one. I thought, "my eyes are playing tricks on me. Maybe I am just bored and getting sleepy." But I knew that wasn't true, I was very interested in what my friend had to say. Nevertheless, I got up, went to the restroom to wash my face with cold water, served colas to my friends, and sat back down. I was wide awake. It didn't take long for the light to reappear.

Having exhausted the physical possibilities, it was now time to enter into the halls of psychology. Was I crazy? No. Was I making it all up? Not likely, after all there was no reason. Then what was it? I didn't have an answer, and that was bothering me. A new idea occurred to me, "maybe I'm not the only one who could see this light."

The thought was exciting. I was ready for camaraderie, for shared experience, for answers. For the first time, I ventured to ask someone else if they also saw the light. Each one said no. Had they ever seen a light around someone's head? No. The wind went out of my sail as quickly as it had come. Given the response I received it was quite a while before I spoke of the light again. Although the experience kept recurring and even began taking on new dimensions of color or size.

It wasn't until I started studying metaphysics that I learned what this is and what it means. I had no idea that this was an intuitive insight that could, and in my case would, be refined and honed to aid thousands of people in their search for wholistic health. At the time I knew little about intuition, and even less about intuitive skills. What I knew about psychics was not complimentary. I was less than a novice, I have to admit for a college graduate I had volumes yet to learn.

*E*ach one of us emanates energy.

How we have fashioned energy, what we have used and left unused, creates vibrational patterns. Part of that vibratory pattern is the residual release from the electrochemical exchanges occurring in the body. In the mid-1900's cameras were invented to photograph this energy as it emanates from living forms. This type of work is called Kirlian photography. The radiation of energy from life forms impresses itself directly on film negatives. This is quite different from commercial photography which reproduces scenes by recording the light reflected off of the people or objects photographed. Kirlian photography requires an absence of external light because it records the light radiating *from* the subject. What is registered on film is auric energy.

When I first saw Kirlian photos I was intrigued. These photos of a hand reminded me of pictures of lunar eclipses where everything is black except the crown of solar flares outlining the moon. The light in the Kirlian photo seemed to emanate from what was obviously a hand. Like the moon's crown, the light seemed to move around the fingers, flaring at the tips. I remember thinking to myself, that's like what I see!

I had no idea that something called etheric energy even existed. But I was learning that there are many planes to our existence, and that if answers are not forthcoming from the physical world they might very well be found by exploring these other ones. All these years I had been seeing beyond the physical sense of sight, perceiving the auras of people, trees, and even furniture. Only now was I learning that this kind of extrasensory perception is an innate part of the mind's ability, an intuitive skill that can be refined as an art. I didn't really appreciate the extent of that skilled artistry until I discovered that what intuitive reporters perceive and describe during an Intuitive Health Analysis is the aura.

What the metaphysician calls the aura, the physicist terms an electromagnetic field. These terms describe the energy emanating from every living thing. Both the physicist and metaphysician desire to understand the field. They define and manipulate the energy. Both attempt to remain objective, apart from the energy so they will not interfere with it. This in fact is the mark of a true scientist. For this reason, a team of a conductor and reporter unite their efforts to give the Intuitive Health Analyses. The conductor serves as the objective scientist, directing the analysis, fielding and asking questions for the person requesting the report, while the reader relinquishes conscious control to the conductor entering a highly developed state of intuitive consciousness where the aura can be perceived, identified, and described. The conductor determines what will be examined and the rerporters gives what is seen.

When the health analysis was being developed in the later 1960's, early researchers wanted to help people answer the questions they had about their health. Initially these were questions of desperation, how to end pain or supply answers medical doctors could not give. By seeking a way to use developed intuitive skills to report on isolated health problems the means to access information about the health condition was discovered. Eventually the information took on the form of the analyses currently provided for those requesting intuitive assessments.

The desire to aid others, provide them with intuitive answers to their questions, help them solve their problems and become whole, continues to be an urgent calling for those who give their time in this labor of love. In fact intuitive reporters and conductors accept no financial reimbursement for their work. This has been true from the beginning. The teams that provide the analyses do so on a volunteer basis, and this produces a consciousness conducive to clarity of intuitive perception. All contributions are made to the organization; there is no conflict of interest for the reporter or the conductor because the element of personal physical compensation is not involved in the work they do.

Through the years, the Intuitive Health Analysis has become a one of a kind, invaluable resource for people all over the world. What it can tell you about yourself is quite amazing. Much of this is owing to the way the information is related. In the early years of refining the Intuitive Health Analysis, a structure was developed that most easily describes anyone's state of health. In its most abbreviated form we say the health analysis examines the mental, emotional, and physical condition of the individual.

The report begins where the disorder begins, in the kind and quality of the person's thinking. What the client first hears is an assessment of his mental condition, the problems both past and present that are disrupting clear thinking and interfering with his or her ability to completely use mental faculties and cultivate mental potential. Here are the seed ideas that set up the emotional and physical conditions for disease. Here are the ideas, concepts and ways of thinking that limit Self. Upon examining the problem patterns, what is needed to resolve them becomes apparent. Suggestions for new ways, healthy ways, of utilizing thought energy are given.

Next how that seed idea matures into the life is described in the emotional condition. Here the more psychological aspects of the person often arise. What began as an idea of insecurity in the mental system for one person becomes in the emotional system a bout of self-pity. For someone else it expresses as jealousy. What started as criticism expresses emotionally as blame in one person and loneliness in another. Greed expresses emotionally as resentment or hatred. Connecting threads, patterns of cause and effect, can be readily seen and suggestions for productive change are given for the emotional system.

Generally speaking these are "negative" patterns of thinking. They push people away from us. They interfere with our sense of well-being. They rob us of peace. And they destroy our Self concept, our relations with others, and ultimately our bodies. I keep thinking the doctors of a century ago who traveled to your home, knew your kids' names and most importantly your hopes and fears, were closer to the truth of health than their modern counterparts who are surrounded by machines and too often only know you as a name on an insurance form and one of many bodies they examine in a day. The difference is astoundingly obvious. In many ways the past is our future, but with the many advantages that we have gained in 20th century science and technology. The mental and emotional assessment of the Intuitive Health Analysis can empower the health practitioner of your choice, in any field, with otherwise immeasurable insight into what is causing your pain and how to alleviate it – permanently.

Finally, the aura of the physical body is examined; detailing any malfunction of systems, organs, or cells. The aura of every system is reviewed as the reader seeks to isolate and describe disorders and their correction. Suggestions for symptomatic relief are given as well as recommendations for appropriate treatments that will alleviate suffering and correct offending conditions. Sometimes what will bring balance is as simple as more sunshine or a chiropractic adjustment or adding a food to your diet. Sometimes what was believed to be the source of a problem is revealed to be the effect of something else or not even a problem at all. Whatever the condition of the physical body, it is reported. And the reports are astounding.

Intuitive Health Analyses enable us to understand the connections between mind and body in ways others are still speculating. This research goes far beyond describing mental processes as "negative" or "stressed". It isolates the exact pattern of thinking that is causing specific malfunctions in the body.

This is phenomenal.

The use of intuition in this fashion portends an inspiring future for humanity as we open ourselves to what connects us to each other, to the world around us, to a common Source. Intuitive Health Analyses are just the beginning of what man will discover about those connections in the next hundred years.

The ideal use of an Intuitive Health Analysis is as a first opinion. They are best understood as given in their entirety for they present a wholistic image of the person. Each analysis reflects its subject. Similarities in universal thought patterns or in the commonalities of body functions are apparent yet no two analyses are ever alike, just as no two people are exactly alike. We all may find benefit from the suggestions given, but the analysis is tailored to restore optimum health for the person receiving the reading.

The best way to become educated is first hand experience, and so we begin a series of analysis transcripts with commentaries by those who requested the information. These are people like you and me, of varied ages, all walks of life and several countries. What they have in common is the desire to know what they can do to ensure a healthy, fulfilling life. Here is what they discovered.

A general awakening comes when the person receiving intuitively-accessed knowledge honestly considers what it reveals about him or her self as you will see through John Clark's eyes. John was in his early thirties when he received his first intuitive report. For years he had been struggling with a chronic condition that very few people knew about although that was not his reason for requesting a health analysis. That reason was addressed in his analysis' opening statements:

> *We see within the mental system there is a great deal of frustration that this one is holding on to mentally. We see much of this is the formation of this one's own ideas as to what this one needs to battle against concerning the environment. We see that there are many ways where this one does try to escape this one' s own responsibilities.*

"When I had this reading I felt a great relief. I felt that I was searching for reasons to follow through with what I had started, reasons I was in situations in my life at that time. I was at that time living with my girlfriend and was very frustrated with the relationship and frustrated with the kind of responsibility I had chosen to take in that situation. I wasn't really sure if I was going to move on in this relationship or if I would be running away from it or if I was doing what I needed to do for myself, so I was caught in my own little mind games and traps of 'should I or shouldn't I?'

> *We see there is a battle which is occurring in that this one is not*
> *responding to what it is that this one does want to accomplish and*
> *does want to do. Would suggest to this one that by making the*
> *environment and what this one considers to be the expectations of*
> *society the scapegoat for the self and the excuse as to why this one*
> *is frustrated with the goals or the lack of being able to achieve those*
> *goals, there will continue to be the frustration that is spoken of.*
>
> *Would suggest to this one that each day this one set out to do*
> *something that this one wants to do solely for the self. Would*
> *suggest that in initiating this, this one could begin to see that there*
> *is the time if this one will cause it to be available to the self. Would*
> *suggest also to this one that this one begin listening to the ways*
> *where this one uses such phrases as what this one "should", "ought*
> *to", "needs to" or "has to" do. Would suggest that in this way this*
> *one is setting outside of the self and away from the self any freedom*
> *because this one is likewise setting aside from the self the respon-*
> *sibility for the action on the part of the self, therefore putting it in*
> *the hands of others. Would suggest doing something this one wants*
> *to do each day will aid this one in understanding that it is to the self*
> *that the responsibility does lie.*

"When I heard this reading it gave me something immediate to practice as far as doing something for myself each day. I was in the midst of carrying some old habits around with me from adolescence that were irresponsible, destructive and not very caring and nurturing to myself. So in order to change some of these habits I decided that instead of putting money into things that weren't going to help me or weren't going to be something lasting or fulfilling, I would spend that money on something that was going to be something I could use; a good piece of clothing, maintain my car, improve the building I lived in.

"In a very short period of time I felt myself start to gain momentum as far as being much more directed, much stronger; stronger will power. I really started to change fast. Things that I had considered big dilemmas were now places where I could make a decision and go with that decision. In doing so I felt great about myself. I felt I was taking my life in my own hands rather than letting someone or something direct me."

We see that concerning the emotional system the resentment and the anger that is oftentimes used to repel others from the self and oftentimes used as a way in which to belittle or chide the self, is also used to motivate the self. Would suggest to this one that as there begins to be the formation of desires and the responding to this, this one will not necessarily need to hold on to the resentment and the chiding...Would suggest that this one replace those areas that this one finds fault with the self with areas of what this one wants instead.

We see within the area of the physical system that there is a difficulty within the stomach area, within the esophageal area and within the small intestines. We do see for the liver to be affected. We see that there is inflammation that is occurring in the esophageal area and within the stomach itself. Would suggest that there be taken into the system that of a sage tea. Would suggest also that this body would benefit from the intake of carbon, also the use of lysine, the use of vitamin B complex. Would suggest the intake of dairy products, particularly the use of buttermilk, the use of yogurt. Would suggest that this one eliminate fried foods, but not to eliminate that of the red meats. We see also that this one could benefit from the use of chewing of the food more completely as it is taken into the system. We see there are times where there is a build up of a gaseous reaction here and would suggest the intake of baking soda diluted with water.

"I also saw in the reading there were places in my mind and in my body that I was unaware of as far as problem areas. I started to figure out how the type of choices I was making were causing my body to fall apart really quickly. Places I wasn't even aware of were becoming areas of concern and so it did wake me up to the need to use what I know about nutrition and to get more exercise, to take care of myself."

We see concerning the area of the liver there is a build up of scarring in this area. We see that this affects the blood vessels within this area. We see that there is some effect upon the major arterial system to this area as well. We see that this is a breaking down. Would suggest that it would be important for this one to become honest in developing a worthiness as to this one's existence and a direction to be taken to fulfill this one's own purpose for existence.

We see that there is some sluggishness within the lymph system. We see the spleen is affected as well. We see the intake of goldenseal would be of benefit to this system. Also increase in water. Would suggest some mild type of exercise which would stimulate the lymphatic areas throughout the body. The use of massage can be of aid in this regard as well. Would suggest the intake of fruit juices particularly that of the citrus fruit juices. We see there is a lacking of potassium within this system. Would suggest that this one would benefit from the intake of bananas.

We see there is some difficulty in the transverse, descending and sigmoid colon area. We see there is a type of scarring where there has been inflammation and ulceration in the shape concerning the descending and the turn of the transverse colon area. Would suggest that the use of calcium, potassium, and phosphorus would be of aid here. Also the use of those foods which are rich in bulk but an increase in the fluids that are taken in at the same time. We see that within the area of the prostate that there is some inflammation within this area. The use of vitamin A, B, C and E would be of aid here. Would suggest that it is important at this time for this one to initiate action as opposed to being a victim of circumstance.

We see within the area of the spinal column there is difficulty in the discs in the 4th and 5th thoracic. We see also difficulty within the cervical, of the axis and 4th cervical, difficulty in the 9th and 10th thoracic. Would suggest chiropractic or osteopathic attention. This is all. (6-1-87-GBM-1C)

"I was aware of digestive upsets, but I attributed them to my chronic condition, not realizing that this was affecting so many parts, stomach, esophagus, liver, colon. I felt very much exposed, exposed to the extent that I was hiding a lot, or at least I thought I was. I was hiding a condition, hiding an illness from others. With the reading I started to open up, to admit and to communicate about where I was, to openly dream about being able to heal myself, to be healed.

"This was a time I began to embrace my learning. I was very anxious to take steps to learn how to be a teacher, to continue and follow through with my learning in this class in metaphysics that I had been in for three or four months. Even though I was very active in my profession as an actor, I just was not stimulated the same as I was when it came to learning about myself, learning how to grow. I appreciated the kind of ideas that stimulated me to follow through on clearness of thinking that started me moving forward and making decisions and changes about who I was going to be and to really get going on them. I became brave and started to really add on to my level of courage in making the kind of choices that were going to really make a difference."

John's story in some ways was just beginning when he received this analysis. It was in many ways the opening of a new chapter of his life. He had taken great pains to hide his diabetic condition from others for years and to deny it in his own thinking. By requesting intuitive analysis John was affirming a new willingness to understand and take control of his physical health as he had refused to do since his diagnosis as a teenager.

Rather than embrace the information and act on the suggestions with a sense of necessity and commitment, John set a new pattern. He would procure an Intuitive Health Analysis, be momentarily inspired – or frightened – into action, and then after days or sometimes months his motivation would wane and he would return to old patterns of thinking and action. After several years, John placed the analyses in the same category as doctors and drugs: when he was in trouble he needed help, a quick fix, be it another drug, surgery, or intuitive identification. What began as a means to change the quality and kind of life he lives fell prey to the same patterns of thinking that produced his ill health originally.

However, John's desire for a different life, however fleeting or undisciplined, has given him knowledge, experience, and hope far beyond the norm. It has tripled his life span enabling him to work, marry, and most importantly learn. It is that desire to learn that continually returns him to Intuitive Health Analysis for that is where he sees a complete picture of himself as a whole being. As a result, John has procured a dozen readings over more than a decade. Although it was not his intent at the time, each successive analysis documents the progression of disease in his body and as such gives invaluable wisdom for those of us who know of someone battling chronic disease or who experience it ourselves. John's story as revealed in his analyses is told poignantly by his wife Dr. Laurel Clark later in this book.

*H*ow each person responds to the information received in an Intuitive Health Analysis is truly individual. Just as the ways in which we are open to instruction vary. Some constantly seek to improve themselves and so they invite sagacious criticism, while others wanting things to remain the same reject it. The grace with which compliments are received or the ingratitude which snubs the bestower, reveals the attitudes often described in these readings. The open-minded, learning individual gains the most because he embraces growth and change. While the latter does best to remember the Biblical counsel, "The truth hurts, but the truth will set you free."

Upon receiving his analysis, John gave it serious thought allowing the information to stimulate him into action. The report encouraged him to use what he had learned about good health through his life, and he now realized some of his aches and pains were the effect of taking that knowledge for granted. He was a little shocked to find out how far-reaching those effects were in his own body. The truth didn't hurt John because the truth was what he wanted and it freed him, if only for a short time. The health analysis offered him direction mentally, resolve emotionally, and physical treatments to pursue.

This was not the case for the marketing specialist from Kansas City. Although she immediately verified the analysis' description of her physical body, she also immediately rejected the mental and emotional descriptions. "It's not me!" she repeatedly declared, virtually ignoring what she didn't like about the information for months. What she did like she told others about, often sharing the details of her analysis.

"The clincher for me," she writes, "was when my mother heard my analysis and responded so strongly. I did not tell her anything about the reading. I simply played it for her. When it was done playing she said, 'I don't know who that person is, but that person just said many things I know about you because I am your mother, however I know you don't see that in yourself. That is remarkable.' Indeed the information was truly transformational."

Once this woman relaxed her defenses, she was able to hear the complete thoughts being conveyed in the report rather than isolated words or phrases. The analysis saying she "didn't listen" was actually *"Would suggest to this one to practice causing the mind to be still and to practice listening for this one does have difficulty in listening to this one's own Self as well as listening to others."* "Being gullible" and "controlled by others" was actually *"this one is very subject to the environment and that due to the lack of control that this one does practice with this one's thoughts, this one is very much influenced by whatever stimuli are around the Self."* She had convinced herself that the analysis was a personal attack when it was not. After all the person giving the analysis did not know her, had never even met her, and so had no bias toward her and certainly no animosity against her. Her ideas of being personally attacked were indeed her own and the first place for her to admit the harmful ideas she herself created and perpetuated.

Getting to the point of hearing her analysis as if it was not about her but about someone else, aided Lori greatly to become objective with the information she had received and put it to good use. "When I first received an Intuitive Health Analysis, I was open to the idea of someone, a total stranger being able to identify the condition of my physical body. I had a vague idea that my mental thoughts and attitudes may be related to my health, but I had not been able to make any clear connection between my thoughts and my physical health. The analysis very clearly did this for me."

One question and answer that exemplifies this is the following:

This entity asks, what is the reason for the sinus congestion?

We see that when this one is scattering the attention, this one does have difficulty in receiving information that is brought to the Self. We see that this one does interpret this as being overwhelmed, when in fact it is not that there are too many experiences within this one's life it is that there is a need for this one to give attention to one thought at a time, to one thing at a time and to one experience at a time. As far as symptomatic relief would suggest the use of acupressure, this would be the area in the brow bone and the inner corners of the eyes. This would relieve the pressure." (2-12-91-BGO)

"When I received my analysis on a cassette tape, I listened to the tape over and over because the information was so revelatory to me. When presented with the physical conditions of my body, it was right on target for what I was experiencing.

"When I heard the mental and emotional attitudes a piece to a puzzle was set in place in my mind."

.....We see a constant scattering of ideas. Because this one has many thoughts, many desires, this one does have difficulty in causing the mind to be still. Would suggest to this one to practice concentration. Would suggest to this one to practice causing the mind to be still and to practice listening for this one does have difficulty in listening to this one's own Self as well as listening to others. Would suggest that with exercise this one could cause the mind to be still but that this would involve this one admitting and practicing that this one is the director of this one's thoughts, therefore, this one can have this kind of control....

We see within the emotional system that this one's emotions fluctuate widely. We see that this one is very subject to the environment and that due to the lack of control that this one does practice with this one's thoughts, this one is very much influenced by whatever stimuli are around the Self. Would suggest to this one to practice separating this one's thoughts from this one's senses. For this one is not even aware what causes the distractions within this one's mind. Would suggest the practice of concentration exercises; would suggest the use of some type of exercise that does stimulate this one to identify this one's senses would aid this one in forming this kind of discrimination.

"These words described things I had 'felt' yet not been able to clearly identify and communicate. Still more of the information became useful to me in later months as I could use and apply the insights given to me on a deeper level. These were insights I may never have discerned on my own.

"I scattered my attention due to fear and emotional outbursts. The reading suggested exercises in concentration, dream interpretation, and meditation. I was able to enroll in a class to teach me these skills. Within three months, through following instructions and taking these classes, I changed my life dramatically. I was able to excel in my career and received considerable notice from my manager and peers. I resolved conflicts I had with my co-workers. I began to sleep restfully at night. I learned to be more attentive, productive, and reason using my new acquired concentration skills.

"I had been under a doctor's care for allergies and painful tension in my jaws. I no longer need medical care or medication after three months of applying the mental and physical suggestions provided to me. This has saved my insurance company and myself thousands of dollars in the past seven years.

Her analysis also allowed Lori to dispel falsehoods accepted as limitations she would have to learn to live with: "I thought allergies were a way of life and that my jaw pain would be something one 'tolerates' as a sign of 'aging.' This absolutely changed my life, inspired me to dream a bigger dream of myself, and be genuinely happy for once in my life."

"I am a Registered Nurse," says Linda Jones, a middle-aged, divorced mother of a grown daughter. Like many people sincerely interested in helping others in need, Linda is devoted to doing everything she can to restore people to good health. Because her work does not provide all the answers to the problems she sees, she is often willing to learn something that will assist her in her work. And like many health practitioners over the years, Linda was quite surprised by the scope and clarity of Intuitive Health Analyses.

"I became a nurse to aid people to become healthy. I found myself at work in the position of 'putting out fires' – taking care of very sick, acutely ill people. Yes, they would get better but nowhere near what I considered to be healthy, happy and productive.

"Here I was, for the most part healthy and productive, yet the year before the reading had been the worst for me as far as health was concerned. I started out getting strep throat then a recurrence of the flu three times that year. I attributed that to an allergy to the flu shot I took that year. I had continual bouts of sinusitis and unless I took Seldane in the morning and Benadryl at night along with other sinus medicine I had a hard time breathing.

"After the strep throat I developed high blood pressure and then had PVC's, (premature ventricular contractions or skipped heart beats) and heart palpitations. Inderal and hydrochlorothiazide were prescribed for that. Then I needed potassium to make up for what the water pill removed. At the point of the reading I could say I was in a state of desperation and open to try anything to get off the medicines. The medicines were just a panacea for the underlying disease process. The more I read and studied the more confused I got about nutrition and exercise and herbs. One philosophy said milk was bad for you and the other said drink it. Another said even vitamin

C could hurt someone. I didn't know what to believe and I wanted some answers which the doctors were unable to give me. They just kept prescribing more and more medicine to cover up the symptoms not a cure. I continued to move farther and farther from the state of health I desired to have.

"At the time of the analysis I was able to be present. I wrote out a list of around thirty questions I had about my health. These people didn't know me. I knew what was going on with me and I wanted to make sure that everything was covered at least physically. I began crossing off question after question as they were answered by the reporter. I only asked seven questions and most of these had been answered in the main part of the analysis."

The body of Linda's first Intuitive Health Analysis given in May, 1986, read like this:

We see within the mental system that there is a form of doubt that is being conjured up by this one. We see this one uses this as a type of insurance in regard to this one's viewpoint as to how this one can fail. We see that in doing so however this one is attempting to keep all bases covered. We see that it makes it difficult for this one to be able to build a trust and respect for the self.

We see that there are times where this one is somewhat secretive as to this one's motives and as to this one's methods and we see that what is produced in this can be of benefit to the self. We see the way it is being approached at this time is through a means of doubting this one's own motives. The use of meditation can be quite beneficial to this one not only in learning how to hear this one's motives but learning how to expand this one's ideas, not to try and live according to the ideas of others but to develop authority in learning from this one's own experiences.

We see that it is quite important for this one to use review as a form of evaluation instead of as a form of justification. We see that in many ways this one tries to reach the past as a means of justifying or as a means of looking for a certain process but we see that instead this one will use this as a way in which to cause a forcing action within the self. Would suggest that this is a beginning for this one. It is a way for this one to determine specifically the image that this one wants to build of the self and [to] use the conditions and circumstances on a daily basis in order to practice this. We see that there is a starting action and then a backing away or a waiting that keeps this one in that state of self doubt. Would suggest instead that this one reach further [ahead] instead of backing away or thinking that there is a need for rest.

We see that in the area of the emotional system there are times when this one causes there to be what would be seen as an evenness in this area but instead it is actually a suppression. We see it is a way that this one fools the self into thinking that there is an element of control. We see there is a desire to understand control at this point but we see the methods this one chooses to do so oftentimes leaves this one quite empty and frustrated. Would suggest to this one that the control can be gained as this one will choose to experiment both in communication and on purpose with the use of the emotions as well as in the communication of this one's thoughts. We see that it is most beneficial for this one to use determination. This can only be achieved when this one is reaching toward something as opposed to holding on to something that is stagnant.

We see within the area of the physical system there is some difficulty within the esophagus and we see that there is some difficulty in the polaris area as well. There is inflammation present within this area. We see for the pancreas to be affected at this time. There would be a benefit to the taking-in of buttermilk and also the use of Jerusalem artichoke.

We see for there to be a fluctuation in the thyroid at this time. We see that there are attempts made of stimulating the rejuvenation of properties that are part of this action here. Would suggest to this one that this would have to do with the stop-start action or the forcing which occurs. Would suggest to this one causing there to be a beginning of an action and the following through, is where this one is already reaching for the next step; as opposed to coming to a point of conclusion and then waiting. There is a need for shellfish and green leafy vegetables.

We see that the use of vegetables would be quite beneficial to the whole digestion and eliminatory system at this time. We see that there is need for an increase in the B complex that is taken into the system, also the use of that of lecithin. We see there is some reaction at this time within the area of the liver. This has some degree of interference in the purification processes of the body and there is an effect that is occurring within the area of the liver. The use of the lemon water would be of benefit and also that of the lecithin that has been recommended. Would suggest that there be increase in the intake of vitamin C and that this be used throughout this one's day. We see that in regards to this area [it] would benefit this one to use honey periodically in this one's diet and to use pineapple juice.

There is a build up of mineral deposits in the kidney and this causes there to be some interference in the filtration process. We do see that because of some imbalances of the hormones there is a dumping of what would be seen as proteins by the system. We see therefore that the use or intake of the proteins is particularly important at this time.

Within the area of the muscular system there is some waste being trapped. Would suggest that the tension and relaxation of the muscle groupings of the body is beneficial to this system as well as the use of visualization – seeing the breaking free of the trappings of certain hormones that have not reached, or been as accessible to, the areas that they were intended.

We see that there is a fluctuation within the heart muscle. There is some corrective action occurring here but there is also some stress that is being placed on this area. We see that this one becomes angered quite easily. This does have an immediate effect upon the circulatory system and the heart as this one will involve the self in blame and forget what it is that this one is seeking to learn or understand. This can be corrected.

We see within the area of the spinal column there is some difficulty in the lower thoracic and lumbar area that would benefit from chiropractic attention. There is also misalignment in the fifth and sixth thoracic and the third and fifth cervical. This is all. (5-10-86-GBM-10)

"Wow! As the reading continued I felt like I was being dissected inch by inch, molecule by molecule. I was taken apart and put back together again in minutes. I learned the **cause** – the mental cause – of the difficulties I had been experiencing. Now all I had to do is to take action on what I heard. I had to prove to myself whether the answers I received were true or not and the only way to do that was to do what the reading told me to do. I first began with the physical symptomatic relief.

"Mentally I needed to be decisive, and to set goals and create what I desire. My oversensitivity to what others said to me had brought on the sinus problems. I needed to be creative in positive ways instead of creating fears and restrictions. Most of all I needed to become useful to the Self.

"Years before, after my divorce I could think of no reason to live except for my beautiful daughter. She needed me, but not as much as I needed her. I began living through her. If she did well, I was okay and if she didn't, I wasn't. What a burden to place on a four-year-old child. I needed to understand the anger and release it. To learn to be at peace with myself.

"Physically, I went out and bought the herbs, vitamins, and minerals suggested. I ate Brazil nuts, shellfish, green vegetables. I had chiropractic attention and massage."

Linda began studying applied metaphysics where she learned how to breathe properly and how to meditate. She also learned how to use the power of her mind to direct life force in the body for vitalization and for healing. "I noticed a huge difference in a month. My sinuses began clearing up and slowly I came off the sinus medicine. Then I began noticing my blood pressure staying on the lower side of normal. During the analysis I wanted to know about the medication for blood pressure I was taking. The conductor asked, 'Are there any suggestions as to what this one can do in order to decrease the medication?' and the reader responded, *'Fulfill this one's own desires, and become responsible for the learning in the process.'* I went to see my doctor and received guidance in coming off the blood pressure medicine. At the end of 3 months, I was off the water pills and potassium and after 6 months I was off all medicines. I was taking herbs, meditating and changing my attitudes instead. I began backing off the herbs by listening to my body.

"I received my second health analysis in 1988. By then I had made many changes in my thinking. I was learning to become responsible for my learning and for my desires. I became a control freak. I went from creating fears and limitations to conjuring up doubt."

> *We see within the mental system that there is a very strong desire on this one's part to be creative and also to be useful. We see this one's difficulty however is in this one being responsible for what this one creates, for what this one does desire. We see because of this, this one will attempt to create fears and attempt to create restrictions – purposefully – so this one can see this action in process. Would suggest however it becomes very much a distracting element in this one's life and in this one's ability to learn.*

We see that in many ways this one looks for struggle as being something that would indicate this one's ability to have confidence within the self. However, we see that this develops a mistrust within the self at this time. Would suggest that this one give attention to how this one causes action physically, also in the action in the mind and in this way to cause learning on purpose from the experience, not after this one has had to go through the ordeal, as this one would see it, of the experience and then assume that there has been some kind of learning. Would suggest to this one that the mistrust occurs because this one does not decide and does not willingly become responsible to the experience and how this one will change regarding using that experience.

Would suggest to this one that decisiveness would be most beneficial at this time for this one to develop, also an image of worthiness regarding the self. We see there is a very strong urge for importance but there is not seen where this one is needed by others to achieve that importance. Would suggest that this one is needed but it would be most beneficial if this one would become important to the self.

"No I hadn't learned how to be positive in my creations yet. I did have quite definite ideas of what I wanted though. I was more decisive. In the area of causing action on purpose I was misusing the past as a means of justifying or finding cause and forcing myself to do things based on the past instead of creating an image of myself that I wanted to live up to and be. It was important for me to follow through on my decisions.

"The way I was dealing with my anger and other emotions was to suppress them. I thought this was keeping me on an even keel and balanced. After all, I didn't explode or get angry as often and I thought I had healed this area. I discovered through the reading that this was not so."

We see within the area of the emotional system that there is a great deal of guilt and fears that this one will build out of proportion. We see that this is done because of this one's urge to create and to become creative. Would suggest that through this there can be equally as much excitement as this one begins to identify those things which this one does have and has experienced and understands. Would suggest that also the guilt be recognized for what it is, a diversion and a way for this one to understand this one's own importance. Would suggest, however, that [not] until this one accepts the learning in these experiences day to day will this one understand the usefulness of the guilt.

We see that there is a great deal of resentment as well and that this is because of this one's attention continually being on the outside or the external situations as being the impetus or stimulation for this one's changes.

Linda comments, "I began learning to express emotions purposefully. This was difficult at first. A more recent analysis said I play with my emotions. I considered at that time that I had come a long way. Now I know how to cause emotions on purpose and to use them effectively. My next step is to learn from the emotion at the time I experience it."

The physical assessment a year and a half later showed some conditions remaining the same while others had changed. The hormonal imbalances described in the first analysis centered on fluctuation in thyroid function. The follow-up reading described the further impact of Linda's indecisiveness, the start-stop action she perpetuated and had yet to change:

We see within the area of the physical system that there is a difficulty in the endocrine system concerning the pituitary, hypothalamus, and the thyroid. We see that these imbalances cause there to be a hormonal imbalance within the system that also causes some difficulty in the way that this body responds to heat and cold...We see that regarding the thyroid, it would be of some relief to take in that of shellfish, and that of the green leafy vegetables, and the use of zinc, calcium, manganese and magnesium, as well as, vitamin B complex would be helpful to the endocrine system as well. Would suggest that regarding the difficulty concerning the pituitary, it would be important for this one to learn how to think or reason rather than to live in the reactions that have been spoken of.

Hormones were still trapped in muscles, with similar recommendations for symptomatic relief:

We see that there has been trapped within the musculatory system some different hormones that cause there to be waste trapped within the musculatory system as well. Would suggest the use of

*Brazil nuts to be taken into the system. Would suggest that this one
involve the self in exercises where this one is tensing and relaxing
the different body groupings independently.*

Linda's efforts to restore her mind and body to health were now causing a
release of energy and waste materials, causing the lymphatic system to work
overtime. Suggestions were given to lighten the burden and ease the strain
in her body's cleansing system:

> *We see within the area of the lymphatic system that there is a build
> up of toxins and waste here. The use of lymphatic massage would be
> most beneficial. The use of goldenseal tea would be helpful and
> niacin in the vitamin B that has been recommended would also be
> helpful in stimulating a flushing action and a cleansing action within
> these areas.*

There were the basic areas covered in the body of the analysis. Linda was
curious about her progress in other areas not mentioned because they were
no longer primary disorders. Her first area of concern was the condition of
her heart and circulatory system. The first analysis had described *"fluctuation
within the heart muscle"* resulting from Linda's anger and tendency to
blame. After a year and a half of striving to redirect her thinking toward
learning and her emotions toward understanding, and of daily meditation
sessions, the analysis found the heart still being burdened:

> *...there is some stress that is being placed upon the area of the heart.
> We see that there has been a build up of some deposits, not only
> within the heart area but within the arterial system as well. We see
> that this causes there to be the fluctuation or difficulty in the
> circulatory system, but the major difficulty in the circulatory system
> is due to the central nervous system and the way that there is
> anxiousness purposefully produced, which has been related. We see
> for symptomatic relief the use of fish oils, garlic, mushrooms,
> sassafras, and ginseng could be of some benefit.*

"For the most part I am in better health now years after my first
analysis than I was in 1986. I take herbs and vitamins occasionally as needed
and I have health analyses done periodically to check my progress. There

are longer and longer periods in which I do not experience sinus difficulties. I have continued to keep my blood pressure controlled without medicines.

"From my own and others' experience I can testify that Intuitive Health Analyses are the most beneficial for healthy people because they aid one to become optimally healthy by learning what the underlying cause is and change it. This causes permanent lasting healing."

Of all the valuable insights she gained in both analyses, Linda still talks about the response she received when she asked for suggestions to aid her to honestly give and receive. The answer was so penetrating that now years later she still finds it profoundly descriptive of how she thinks and lives. She is ever grateful that the analysis brought it to her attention for it has enhanced her understanding of herself and deepened her relations with others:

> *Would suggest to this one that this one's action of giving oftentimes is not giving but is trying to create a dependency upon herself of others; therefore, having some way to receive by there being a need of the self by others. Would suggest to this one that this one place the attention upon giving as being an action whereby this one is offering something of the self for the purpose of offering it. Not for the purpose of what it will create in another, but [for the purpose of what it will create] in the self. Would suggest likewise that in receiving this one see that the difficulty in receiving is associated with [what] this one creates in accordance with this one's desires as opposed to this one's fears. (1-7-88-GBM-10)*

Sharing what you learn in an analysis with those closest to you can speed your healing.

They can support your efforts toward change and gain understanding of why you are like you are. This can open new lines of communication, deepening your association. A true friend, one who has your best interest in mind, can be a powerful healing force in your life as computer programmer John Harrison discovered.

"When I received my first health analysis I was getting it to check on my state of health after an attack of diabetes. I expected to receive a physical report. I was shocked when it started out talking about how I was avoiding responsibility."

We see within this one there is a fear of responsibility. We see that this one desires responsibility in that this one desires to be important, this one desires to make a contribution, but this one views responsibility as something constricting and entrapping, and therefore, this one shies away from opportunities to increase this one's skill level, experience level, talents and understandings. Would suggest to this one that there is a need for this one to expand this ones idea of responsibility to go beyond the idea that there is something expected of this one by others to the idea that increased responsibility means increased understanding, experience and freedom for this one. Would suggest that this one admit to the Self that there is a desire for expanded experience and for this one to respond to this.

"My first thought was, 'Where did that come from? I didn't pay for this. Let's get back to physical problems.'

"I knew I had been avoiding responsibility. The analysis said I thought responsibility was a burden. It pointed out that I desired freedom and that responsibility could provide me with that freedom. The reading explained that by putting myself into positions of responsibility, I would have the freedom to do more things."

"The one thing the analysis left out was my ability to avoid confronting problems in my life. This is where my teacher in the School of Metaphysics stepped in since she was committed to my soul growth and development, she continually challenged me to confront my limitation to responsibility." By trusting someone, in this case a teacher, John was acting upon the counsel in his analysis:

We see within the emotional system that this one is somewhat reserved emotionally and this one views the emotions as something private and personal and therefore, does not share his emotional experiences with others. We see that at times this produces a kind of sadness for we see that this one does desire inwardly to share the Self with others but consciously keeps the Self away from this. Would suggest that this one choose particular individuals to share the Self with and by gradually doing this with particular individuals, this one can then expand this to include all people which will aid this one in changing the loneliness and the isolation to experiences of joy and peace. (2-20-96-LJC-1)

John's choice of his teacher as a confidante was a wise one. He describes his teacher's vigilant instruction: "This loving assault on my limitation broke down my resistance enough for me to intuitively receive the second reason why I was avoiding responsibility. I didn't want to be in a position where I could hurt someone. My teacher then went to work on showing me how I could use it to help people. I decided that in order to become the person I wanted to be I would have to quit running from it and embrace it.

"Today I am not wild about taking on responsibility. I don't run as fast away from it like I used to. I do take on a lot more of it and have begun to notice the pain I cause myself in my life when I avoid it. Embracing change is the key to enjoying life along with creating a purpose for that change. The analysis helped bring to my conscious mind a major obstacle to my being happy and free. It pointed out the positive benefits of embracing and using what I was avoiding to help me to receive what I desired."

In light of what John learned about himself, and how he was able to use the information to enhance his life, the physical part of the analysis faded in its importance to him. This report described a *"swelling in the heart muscle, high blood pressure, and restriction in the circulatory system"* as well as addressing stiffness in the joints of the body, spinal misalignments, urinary tract infections, and prostate problems.

A second analysis just seven months later revealed the effort John was putting forth for there was some progress in all areas. But what concerned John the most was the diabetic condition. And this is one of the most common uses of the Intuitive Health Analysis: the detailed screening of how the energies of the body are being used, abused, or misused, and what can be done to replenish and redistribute them. The physical part of John's analysis began by describing the condition of his endocrine system, including the pancreas:

> *We see within the physical system there are imbalances within the nervous system and the endocrine system. We see that there is a incrustation that is beginning to appear in the pituitary. We see that there is slight swelling in the right side of the thyroid. We see that there is restriction in the pancreas and its functioning. We see that there is restriction also in the adrenals. We see that there is a need for the change in the way that the thinking is used as has been*

described. This one needs to reason much more and to direct the action of the imagination consciously. This would aid in stimulating the action of the pituitary and would release the incrustation that is beginning to build around it. We see that this in turn would ease much of the nervous disruption and it would aid in a greater flow of emotional energy into the body and the flow of the energy from and to the senses. We see that the direction of the attention upon what is at hand would aid the body greatly. This one can deny the physical part of the Self very easily and it is very important for this one to appreciate the physical and the body. Would suggest that any kind of activity, a sport or dance where this one would, out of necessity, direct the attention upon moving the body and appreciating the movement itself would be of great assistance in this one beginning to change his opinion of his body and therefore, to change to the image of health this one holds and therefore, the quality of the health of the body itself. We see that there is a need for vanadium in the body; there is a need for chromium. These would aid in the functioning of the digestion and it would compensate for some of the disorders in the pancreas...

This part of the report went on to describe other digestive and eliminatory disruptions and suggestions for their relief.

The mental and emotional attitudes described in this analysis were like continuations of those identified in the first report. The *fear of responsibility* identified initially in the mental system and the tendency toward *emotional reserve* which fueled *isolation* and *loneliness* took on a whole new meaning in the context of the second analysis which dealt head on with how those fears had been dominating John's self-concept and his life:

We see a high level of lack of confidence that this one perpetuates within the Self. We see that there is much this one has to offer other people and indeed wants to, but this one has not disciplined the Self to place the Self in appropriate conditions for the gifts to be given. We see rather this one has allowed the imagination to be undisciplined and therefore, this one has perpetuated false ideas of insecurity in himself of unworthiness and of rejection, which in reality have not occurred.

We see that in reality when this one has given most of the time it has been well received by others, it has been embraced by others and this one has even been encouraged by others. Yet, this one has not acknowledged it and denied it, therefore, has perpetuated this one's loneliness, this one's selfishness and this ones sense of being rejected by others. Would suggest that it is time for this one to recognize that it is of his own making, that it is through the power of his own thinking that this one has created the kind of isolation and loneliness which he often experiences. There is no reason for this one to perpetuate this. There is no cause for it and it does not produce anything that is valuable to himself and to other people.

We see that there is a great need for this one, and this one is becoming more aware of it, of being able to put to use the skills and talents that this one has and to refine these and to add upon them. It is very important for this one to challenge himself in the present. It is important for him to set his ideals high and to strive for them without fail. It is very important for this one to be able to recognize the sense of power, the sense of discipline, the sense of dedication, and loyalty, which this one often finds lacking toward himself and would like to have demonstrated toward himself. Would suggest that if this one wants other people to be certain ways toward him then the easiest and most expedient way to accomplish this is to be those things himself. This is the place for this one to start initiating the kind of change of consciousness which would bring this one what this one has desired...

John was ready to hear this. He had spent months actively working on himself. New thoughts had arisen in his mind and old thoughts had become more pronounced. This analysis accentuated this, like holding a magnifying glass to what is already seen so its composition can be studied. The detail with which the patterns of thoughts are described is quite astounding. The more reflective and Self-aware the individual requesting the analysis, the more easily report are the attitudinal patterns.

John was in his mind too familiar with the state of the art medical response to diabetes. Following the regimen forced him to make physical changes, and mental and emotional ones. But Western medicine didn't answer the question that kept burning in his mind, "Why me?"

John knew from his first experience that the Intuitive Health Analysis was a place where he could ask why and expect an answer. So in his second analysis John asked, "What was the situation that stimulated the attitudes that have led me to the manifestation of diabetes?" The answer was forthcoming:

> *We see that it is the holding onto, the imaging and holding onto,*
> *the insecurity that has been spoken of. This action in and of itself*
> *is one of selfishness and therefore, takes from him the manifestation*
> *of this one's assignment for living, this one's purpose for existence.*
> *It does steal from those in this one's environment because this one*
> *does not give what this one is capable of. (11-8-96-CM-1)*

Verification of the analysis by a medical doctor eases some people's minds.

And quite a few physicians around the globe have not only read or listened to Intuitive Health Analyses at the behest of their patients but copies of analyses are often included among patients' medical records. The most readily obtainable is x-ray confirmation. Subluxated spinal vertebra are seconded by osteopaths, teeth and gum irregularities are confirmed by dental x-rays. More sophisticated, and costly, technology such as CAT scans and MRIs have duplicated the findings reported in Intuitive Health Analyses.

Karen Low, an entrepreneur from Dallas, describes her experience this way. "In December, 1995, I was diagnosed with three fibroids in my uterus. Soon after that exam, I requested an Intuitive Health Analysis, in which I asked about the fibroids, the presence of which was confirmed. I asked the cause of the fibroids and was told:

> *This is also a manifestation of the anger and the harshness that*
> *this one has towards the self, specifically in regard to the ways that*
> *this one has been angry with the self in this one's relationships with*
> *men. Would suggest to this one that this one learn how to love the*
> *self and to practice this and cause this daily. (12-19-95-CM-1)*

I found it very interesting that there were three fibroids, and I had experienced three long-term unhappy or unfulfilling relationships with men.

"In September I had another analysis done in anticipation of my annual gynecological examination. This one told me that there was fibroid tissue in the breast area and in the uterus. I then realized that for a while I had been experiencing a pulling sensation deep in my left breast, and recognized that must be the location of the fibroid tissue.

"When I went to my gynecological exam, I took a copy of the health analysis with me. Before he examined me, I showed my doctor the paragraph in the report that indicated there was fibroid tissue in my breast as well as my uterus. I also told him about the pulling sensation I felt in my left breast. He was very skeptical about the reading. I asked him to simply consider the information as he examined my breasts.

"After the breast examination, he told me he didn't feel anything unusual, and he didn't think there was anything there. However, since I had just turned 40 years old, he said that I needed to have a baseline mammogram done anyway, and that would reveal the presence of any fibroids.

"Before my doctor left the examining room, and much to his chagrin, I requested that he place the copy of the health analysis in my medical file. He argued that the file was only for medical records. I advised him that as far as I am concerned, an Intuitive Health Analysis is a medical record. He placed the report in the file.

"A week later he called me and told me that the mammogram had identified a fibroid nodule in my left breast.

"I greatly appreciated the information given to me in the health analysis. Even though my doctor says that fibroids are "natural" and non-malignant, he says they bear watching. Although the doctor probably would have had the mammogram done anyway because of my age, without the mammogram, he would not have known of the presence of the fibroid tissue in my breast except for the information from the health report.

"Although he says the fibroids will continue to grow until I reach menopause, I intend to use the suggestions in the health analyses to heal myself of this problem. My doctor will be examining me every six months, so it should be easy to chart my progress. I'll keep you informed on the results."

Those who rely upon a medical doctor as their health authority expect that professional to support their seeking other opinions. This does not always happen. Doctors who bear the burden of life and death choices are often disinclined to experimentation. Their prescriptions must be followed as given for that is how they have known them to work in the past for most people. They believe trying a different treatment will result in the loss of valuable time, taking herbs or even vitamins may interfere with the drugs they've prescribed, or like this woman's doctor that for any health information to be valid it must come from a source he is familiar with. That may sound a bit self-centered but when you rely upon someone else as the authority for the condition of your health, you expect them to be certain. Most of the time they are not because they cannot be.

Intuitive Health Analyses do not have all the answers either. What they do have is the capacity to educate and thereby empower each individual to think and act in ways that will produce health. The authority moves from someone or something else to you. You decide. You learn. You change. You heal. You grow. You become the person you've always imagined yourself to be. When you need help, you enlist the aid of others who can offer assistance, guidance, expertise. You have the authority and you have the responsibility. Health analyses encourage the former and make the latter easier to understand.

In my many years of research, what has proven enlightening to me is realizing how technological advances attempt to duplicate the workings of the human mind. This is man's way of seeking certainty in his world. The latest medical machines produce three dimensional pictures for doctors to study. These physical reproductions enable those who perform surgery to see what the intuitively skilled directly perceives. This is also true of a healer. A healer uses his mind – his intelligence and wisdom, the energy and even substance of thought itself – to perceive, evaluate, create, and restore healthful balance in his patient. As we see a progressive increase in the number of people who can heal we will see a proportionate decrease in the number of these machines.

There have been times when people have spent months undergoing extensive technological testing in an effort to diagnose the cause of a problem only to find no answers. This does not mean the pain doesn't exist nor unfortunately does it make that pain go away. It does mean the root of their suffering is not detectable by these means. The Intuitive Health Analysis identifies the cause.

Consider this information concerning what causes tinnitus, the sudden onset of an incessant low grade sound that medical science has yet to explain. Although personal to him, the analysis does reveal the universal cause of this condition. A gentleman asked "what causes the incessant ringing in my ears?" The response referred him to information given in the body of his reading concerning the condition of his nervous system:

> *...There is great difficulty in utilizing the senses fully. We see that there is a significant drop in the electrochemical movement to the auditory system, and to the visual system. We see that in large part this is due to the denial of the emotions that have been spoken of and this one pulling back and away from life experiences. In order for the body to change, this one will need to find a renewed willingness to look and see, to hear and listen, in the experiences. (4-17-93-1-BGC)*

The emotional denial is one way to describe what Dr. Daniel Condron lists in Permanent Healing as the mental cause for tinnitis: "refusal to hear the thoughts of Self". The analysis had earlier described this gentleman's refusal in this way:

> *...We see that emotionally this one becomes stagnant in what this one would identify as approval or rejection. We see that in reality however this is a way for this one to deny his own standards of accomplishment, his own code of ethics, his own ideas of morality. It is much easier for this one to both live up to as well as fail to live up to these codes of standards as long as this one believes they belong to someone else and not him. Would suggest to this one however that this one's thinking creates the self. It is the identity of the self. Therefore whatever code of ethics or standards that this one has entertained, even when this one has tried to put them off on someone else, is his own. Whatever this one has lived up to this one has earned – this one has made a part of the self and will benefit from. Whatever this one has not adhered to, this one has not fed the self and will not have this to draw upon. This is the honesty (in the mental system) that has been spoken of.*

This man could immediately understand what the intuitive report described. He was able to respond to his analysis with life-changing ways of life. His line of business had been in conflict with his own beliefs for years thereby creating inner conflict. He got out of the business, initiated long postponed projects and began new ones. The new ways of thinking did not totally release him from the incessant ringing in his ears but it has significantly lessened, enabling him to think more clearly and sleep better at night. As he says anyone who has experienced this condition knows, this is a Godsend.

Lack of medical diagnosis has been a common reason people first pursue an Intuitive Health Analysis, but increasingly another reason is moving to the forefront: autonomous insight. People want to know what they can do to take control of their health. They want specialized insight not generic textbook descriptions. They want natural ways to be healthy. They want to *permanently* restore balance in mind and body rather than have temporary, symptomatic relief for a condition that still exists or will return. This is the area where the Intuitive Health Analysis is outstanding.

Many people look at Intuitive Health Analyses as others consider yearly visits to a medical doctor a necessary part of life. There is no doubt that the intuitive analysis gives information beyond what medical science affords. For this reason increasing numbers of people assume a balanced approach to health maintenance. Consider Terryll Nemeth's experience.

"I had my first health analysis from the School of Metaphysics in April, 1986. I had been experiencing recurring sinus infections, blood vessels breaking in my eyes, popping in my ears, shortness of breath and a nervous stomach from increasing fear and a sense of foreboding. I felt like my body was falling apart. I went to aerobics and did some weight training regularly so to look at my exterior, I looked like a picture of health, but something was very wrong.

"I had a very good job as an electronics engineer with the Federal Government, a condo, and money but I was still unfulfilled. I had began experiencing much unknown fear and had difficulty being happy with the responsibilities of life. I wasn't sure how this breakdown of my identity and spirit had come to such a head, but I believe I had not learned to cope with the break up of my marriage. In fact, I blamed myself for having made what I termed the big mistake of marrying Matt in the first place. I did not realize it before I had the analysis, but later came to recognize how negative I had become in my thinking."

We see that in the mental system this one has many perverted ways of thinking. We see that a part of this is due to some brain damage that this one has caused. We see that a part of this is also due to this one's own hatred and we see that this one has much difficulty in relating to life as it is.

We see that this one has some very destructive ideas. We see that this one has much difficulty in being responsible for this one's own self without causing detriment to this one's self and others. We see that there is need for this one to begin changing these attitudes, for we see they are not only destroying this one, but are creating a great deal of karma in most unpleasant ways for this one. Would suggest to this one that what this one has considered to be desirable and perverted manners do need to be rethought. Would suggest to this one that this one's emotions have developed the habit of becoming excited only with detrimental emotions such as anger, fear, denial, greed, harm and so forth.

We see that this one has much difficulty in relating to the more beautiful things in life. We see that this one has much difficulty in recognizing much light and in recognizing any truth any more. We see that this one has chosen dishonesty and perversion as this one's thrill and way of life. Would suggest to this one that it is this one's choice what this one does, but would suggest to this one to remember that this one is also the one who experiences and will experience the consequences.

We see that the physical body is having much difficulty at the present time. We see that there are small blood vessels all over the body that are breaking. We see that this one is developing emphysema and this one is experiencing a cancerous condition in the pancreas.

We see that there is a kind of yellowed substance which is a type of infection that acts differently from most infections which is attacking the brain stem, surrounding the brain stem and we see that this is affecting the ears to some extent. We see a similar substance is beginning to form around the liver. We see that some of the components of this infected substance are some of the same components that are found in fat, body fat.

We see some of the blood vessels to also be breaking in the eyes.

We see that the calcium is being used up in this body. There is a need for large intakes of potassium, calcium, magnesium, iron, manganese. We see that there is a deficiency of vitamin A in this

*body, but the body will hardly accept vitamin A, and it does produce
a strong reaction in the body because it is so needed by it. This is
all. (4-29-86-BGO-1M)*

"After receiving that first analysis, I was shocked. I was experiencing conditions of emphysema and worse, cancer. I did not understand the reference to perverted thinking at the time, but I did relate to the fact that I was having difficulty living life, and most of the physical symptoms described in the reading I could relate to.

Terryll was stunned. She immediately sought counseling. "I called my [metaphysics] teacher and she arranged a meeting with her teacher and supervisor. It was pointed out to me that I was killing myself in a variety of ways. I needed to decide if I wanted to live or die. What did I want?

"I decided I wanted to live and started the healing process.

"My counselor, Dr. Laurel Clark pointed out that I had gotten in the habit of stuffing my emotions and that this was unhealthy and growth-limiting. I knew this was true. I judged myself harshly, and to keep from making mistakes I had decided limiting my expression was best. I then recognized that way of thinking as being perverted. So this was one of the ways of thinking the analysis pointed out that was detrimental.

"As a result of learning to still my mind and recognize my thinking, I also realized I had created a habit of thinking negatively. Thinking of the worst case scenario first. Bingo, another perverted way of thinking became visible.

"By creating new brain pathways through the use of concentration exercises practiced daily, and strengthening this concentrated mind through daily experience, I learned to create more positive ways of thinking. I healed my physical body, while I learned to heal my mental attitudes and imaging, using the Kundalini energy, our creative energy which I learned about in classes in Applied Metaphysics in the School of Metaphysics.

"I learned how to change my thinking and how to express my emotions more productively within the year period of time between my first and second health analyses. I had some very profound healing experiences in which I got in touch with the understanding I have in healing as brought out in the analysis. The conductor had asked the reporter if the cancer in the pancreas was reversible at the present time and the reporter stated, *'This one could reverse it and could live.'* My teacher stated that this indicated that

I had understandings in regard to healing that I could draw out of me this lifetime and use these understandings to heal myself. This statement bolstered my spirits and I used it to enhance my belief that I could heal myself. During a healing experience, I knew the cancer was no longer in my body, the thing I was unsure of was how I knew this.

"Eleven months had passed and I determined that it was time for another analysis to gauge my progress. I believed the cancer was no longer present in my body, and I no longer experienced the symptoms described in the first one."

The next analysis confirmed Terryll's belief and reported on her progress. Physically the infection was still present now centered in the colon and stomach, and the lymphatic system was carrying on a valiant effort to rid the body of the invader. A need to purify the lungs of excess mucus and toxins existed but the condition was no longer described as emphysematic. The circulatory system also needed further cleansing but pressure in the capillary system that had caused breaking blood vessels had been eased. No mention was made of the pancreatic condition or of malignancy. What had come so quickly, had eroded just as fast. A sluggishness in the thyroid which was nonexistent a year before was now apparent. Suggestions for further change were given for all areas noted.

Terryll had spent the past year engaged in thought-transforming activities. Daily concentration and meditation exercises had brought flexibility back into thinking. As a result of her desire for wellness and her willingness to change, new light was shed in the second analysis on the construction of Terryll's thought processes. These details about her thinking enabled her to see how she made her recovery more painful than necessary. The attitudes sabotaging her sincere efforts to heal were clear:

> We see for this one to be refusing to listen to this one's own inner thoughts, particularly those regarding this one's own inner authority. There is a need for this one to give more attention to meditation, and receiving from this one's higher Self.
>
> There is a need for this one to pay attention and to get honest with the fact that this one is reacting to all authority figures within this one's life as well. And for this one to begin learning to cooperate with the inner and outer authority in order to know balance within the Self...

We see this one is flitting from one extreme to another at the present period of time due to the refusal to listen to this one's own inner Self and to cause balance within the conscious and subconscious minds...

We see that there is a need for this one to recognize that in this one's adolescent attitudes there is a turning against the good for the whole. We see that there is a need for this one to stop being malicious to regard to this one's own attitudes towards those who are somewhat different than this one at the present time, or in a different position. We see that there is a need for this one to draw forth this one's own love and compassion to deal with this one's Self as well as others, and to begin removing this cloud of resentment from this one's eyes so that this one can pursue the goals that this one does have...

We see that this one's emotionalism needs to be directed in the direction of this one's goals rather than them being a distraction to them....(3-17-87-CR-1M)

Terryll so valued the information she received that she uses Intuitive Health Analyses almost yearly as a means for self-discovery and to promote wholeness and well-being. "The health analyses I have received from the School of Metaphysics down through the years have aided me to reach for greater and greater health. From 1986 to 1995, I received eight analyses. These analyses have proven to be a way to seriously and accurately chart and cause individual growth when used. They helped me to zero in on limitations in my thinking and address these immediately with suggestions by the reporter that promote mental, emotional, and physical healing. Each health report provides the individual with a particular quality of thinking that needs to be changed to cause the Self to be more healthy or heal.

"With most of the analyses I received, I was excited because the information communicated to me that I was making progress in my quest for wholeness. Because I used this information, I noticed in most cases that the next health analysis I received gave more specific details regarding a limited way of thinking than the one previous to it. Each successive Health Analysis gave me a way to see limitations in my thinking from a different perspective. These health reports have allowed me to more easily discover the core thoughts, or the cause for misunderstandings so that I could make productive changes thereby creating growth. With the analyses, I feel as though I am peeling away outer expressions and thinking that no longer serve me as if I were peeling layers off an onion. Revealing the core of the onion is like revealing the core of my soul or subconscious mind.

"In the second analysis I received, the report made reference to a tendency to be judgmental in regard to self and others and to blame others instead of taking greater responsibility: the *maliciousness* and need for *compassion*.

"Amazingly enough, I found out from the third health analysis I received a couple of years later that the criticalness or criticism of myself and others was caused by a laziness in regard to my use of imagination. The report communicated that because I did not imagine enough, I entertained fear or insecurities. This gave way to a defensiveness because I thought I needed to defend my ideas and excuses, instead of directing my thinking forward and so that I manifested my ideals. The next step was a type of blame or criticism or excuses where I misjudged what was actually occurring, thereby distorting my ability to put things into proper perspective.

"Identifying the cause of the criticalness, defensiveness and blame, gave me a way to recognize the habitual patterns in my thinking and change them. I have not yet learned everything there is to using my imagination better, however, I have improved some so that I am not as defensive or critical. I have improved my ability to use proper perspective, and thereby my ability to create.

"I identified from the 1986 health analysis that I cling to ideas about myself that are from an earlier time period. I have not always brought myself up to date in assessing the level of experience I have gained and adding this to the identity that I form about myself. I know I improved on this thereby gaining a clearer perspective, however, I did not make it a part of myself. It reappeared in the last report I had in 1995.

"The next analysis in 1990 revealed that I had taken some steps to reform my perception of myself. The main mental attitude was frustration surrounding my quest to build a new identity. It revealed that I was having difficulty fashioning an identity that I would find pride and respect in. New information came in the form of how I could release these old patterns of thinking. I was told that it would benefit me to begin to separate those ideas which I was taught, and those ideas which *"This one has created and has caused to be her own."* The analysis stated that living with these many different thoughts, some of which I did not claim, caused there to be frustration and confusion, and this in turn caused there to be difficulty in my being able to have true perception. It also stated that this jumble of thoughts caused me to become prejudiced and judgmental in regards to the self and others. This aided me to see how I could also change the judgmental tendency that has been pointed out in the two previous readings.

"I became very excited as I worked with my health reports, because I could very easily see that as I continued to take steps in causing my growth, I earned the right and awareness to recognize, receive, and use cause to continue growing.

"All of the analyses gave me the information that I need to transform the way I create by improving my use and understanding of imagination (reasoning), along with productive use of memory. They also informed me of how I had a need to transform my identity and perception, and use the power of my emotions productively and expansively. The last report I received seemed to tie the transforming of my thoughts and identity together with my desire to fulfill my ideals. I knew there were certain physical things that I had always seemed to create easily at times. However, there were things like the ideals to teach large classes, direct large number of students in the schools I directed, and having fulfilling relationships with men. I found it difficult to have these ideals manifest in my life. I had come to the conclusion, while analyzing my thoughts in this regard, that I had not truly received the idea into myself that my thoughts create and draw circumstances and people of corresponding desires to me. The report helped me to see in what ways I needed to change my thinking to develop understanding in this matter. It stated that I need to imagine what I want, not only physically, but in regard to the state of being that I want to have. It seems I have much experience imaging physical results and causing them to occur, but that now I need to apply this to imaging the way of thinking that I want to have and cause it to occur. The analysis did talk about the conclusion I had come to stating that I was very attached to the idea that I had little control over what I think and that I know this is not true.

"Once again, I am called upon to sort through the thoughts I have to bring myself up to date with the experiences I have had physically, proper perspective and use these to aid in my mental maturity. This analysis has tied together many pieces of information I received in earlier ones. I can see that the ideals I have had difficulty bringing about are ideals that are dependent upon my changing the way I am thinking and fully embracing the power of thought."

Wheneverhealthconcerns are important in your life, regular Intuitive Health Analyses are a welcome addition to and in some cases replacement for yearly visits to a medical practitioner.

Parents often request Intuitive Health Analyses for their young children.

The peace of mind it can bring is immeasurable. Most discover the immense benefit for themselves as a by-product of requesting the analysis rather than the reason for it. In other words, most parents have questions about their child: why is John inattentive at school, does he have attention deficit disorder; why does Jane refuse to play with children her own age, is this retarding her social skills; what causes tantrums, bedwetting, rashes, allergies. Parents are concerned about their child's health in a wholistic way. They want to know about the physical things but they also want to know what's going on in the child's mind. What is he or she thinking? An intuitive analysis gives parents the feedback they are seeking and much more. No one understands this better than my colleague Dr. Pam Blosser.

A graduate of the Maria Montessori Institute in London, Dr. Pam has taught adults and children for over ten years.   When people write to the School of Metaphysics concerning our intuitive consultations, she is the one who receives the requests, schedules them, and directs volunteers to respond in a timely manner. During the summer she directs College Preparatory Camp, a summer camp for young adults held on the campus of the College of Metaphysics. She also mentors *First Teacher*, a spiritual initiation session designed especially for parents. All of these experiences make Dr. Pam uniquely qualified to describe the familial benefits of children's health analyses. Here are some of her thoughts, printed with permission from *Thresholds Quarterly, Vol. No. XX.*

"I have often thought that disciplined, mentally and emotionally healthy children are one of the most delightful sights to behold. They have a curiosity as well as a respect for life and those around them. This does not just happen. Although the child is naturally curious he can quickly have it squelched out of him by the attitudes of the adults around him. As an adult you have the duty to aid children to develop a sense of self control as well as a sense of freedom to explore and discover what life is all about.

"Children are souls in little bodies. When born they are functioning from subconscious mind. They look at life from the soul's perspective. Yet they are in the process of feeling at home in the new vehicle they have chosen, their physical body, and developing the outward thinking patterns in the conscious mind. Their brains and conscious minds are ready and open to receive the stimuli of their environment. It is very important at this time to give children a place to focus, to bring their attention out into the physical. That is why colorful mobiles float above a baby's crib or why there are objects of different textures available for him or her to touch. This aids young children in isolating their attention into one of the five senses. Have you ever wondered why babies tend to put everything in their mouths? It is their way of exploring the physical environment around them, placing another piece of information in their brain for the conscious mind to use in the future.

"Although children are in the process of gathering information in their brains and building their conscious minds, they are still functioning from their subconscious minds. They are receiving the thoughts and emotions of those around them. While in the process of building an identity separate from their parents they are still very much connected to their parents' thoughts. Bringing the attention outward through the senses gives the child a place to develop a sense of autonomy, physically separate from those around him. With any outward experience they can identify the impression of the experience as separate from themselves. The puppy's fur is soft. The puppy and the way it feels is separate from me. Mommy is feeling sad. Mommy and her feelings are separate from me.

"Parents or adults can aid children by directing their attention toward objects or people. Talking, singing or making sounds to the child is an effective way to aid them in bringing their attention into the physical. This means communicating what you and the child are experiencing, have just experienced or are about to experience and what you think and feel about it. Asking them to communicate their experience and thoughts about it gives them the opportunity to express their thoughts and feelings as valid and separate from yours. Any sensory stimulation gives children an opportunity to draw their thinking outward. This is the beginning of the child learning how to use the physical existence more productively and even the beginning of teaching goal setting. Setting a goal gives anyone a place to reach.

Anytime you stimulate a child's attention he must reach out into his physical existence to experience and then bring back into himself a conclusion or judgement about that experience.

> *We see that emotionally this one is bombarded by the emotions of the ones around the Self and this one has no defense for it. We see that this confuses this one. We see that it is not an awareness of confusion but it is a confused state and we see that it does not aid this one in terms of this one's ability to respond easily to the environment. Would suggest that there be tactile exercises for this one, objects that this one can actually feel physically as well as see and hear. As many of the senses as can be used would be of benefit in bringing this one's attention outward and this would aid this one in building some sense of identity and autonomy apart from the environment.   (2-4-92-4-BGC-1M)*

"As the child learns to direct the attention into the physical it is important not to overload her with stimuli but to teach her to hold the attention on a single activity for a prolonged period of time. This would be the beginning of concentration. Here there are many opportunities to build concentration. Direct the child to complete activities. Go for leisurely walks taking time to watch animals, to examine the grass or flowers. Read a story. Draw a picture. Sing a song. Have the child be your assistant in one of your projects making sure you complete it. These activities give the child a chance to slow down her mind and learn through concentration the beauty of creation from start to finish.

"Above all, the best way to aid the child to develop a healthy mental and emotional sense of being is, for you, the adult, to continue to improve your own thoughts and emotions about yourSelf and life. Children have you as their models not only in your actions but in the way you think. They reach to be like you as they grow up because you represent adulthood to them. This doesn't mean you must be perfect. It means being open to change and growth and striving to live up to your ideals. A suggestion in a reading given to parents was:

> *...they tend to be over conscientious at times in terms of their own doubts and fears in relationship to their ideals of parenting. Would suggest that this is a waste of their time and it does take away from*

the joy and the excitement and the discovery of being able to guide this one through the existence. Would suggest that these ones make the change by removing the attention from the doubts or fears and directing the full attention upon who this one is, who they are and how the interaction that they desire can transpire. (3-3-92-3-BGC-1M)

"Life is full of discoveries, and having a child is one of the best ways to learn about life as creation. Guiding another soul, with discipline and love is a duty to be held with greatest awe and respect. As you aid another to unfold you are causing an unfolding in yourSelf as well leading to healthy individuals and healthy relationships. Viewing children as souls desirous of becoming productive adults gives you the freedom to nourish their growth with discipline, keep high expectations of them and appreciate them as unique individuals with unique expressions."

The scope of what is covered in an Intuitive Health Analysis is staggering.

Some questions are mundane, tied to the physical trappings of modern life. Like the person who asks, *"Do you see coffee intake being detrimental to this body?"* For someone savvy on the topic of caffeine the response is probably not surprising:

We see that it does create some pressure in the nerves when this one is failing to relax. It does create a physical condition where this one is trying to offset physical fatigue when in reality this one needs mental adjustments that the release of denial, particularly, that would free much of the energy mentally, emotionally, and physically. Would suggest that this one be aware of how this one is using this substance. (9-15-92-BGC-5)

This question and answer however are by no means generic for in another analysis performed the same day the answer to a similar question from another person is a simple *"No."* Time and again this kind of detail directly pertinent to the individual being assessed appears in analyses.

Some questions are the kind we all ask at one time or another. For instance reproductive questions, whether from a male or a female, are quite common. One woman states she experiences a type of dull headache prior to menstruation. The response reiterates the information already given in her analysis concerning mental struggles for independence and conflicts about her importance, and emotional doubts that lead to both dependencies and defensiveness:

> *We see that this is a variety of physical reactions most of these are in regards to the nervous system. The difficulties in the head that have already been given. Part of it is due to hormonal changes that occur in the action of the pituitary. Would suggest to ease the conflicts within this one mental and emotionally would be of great assistance. (4-17-93-BGC-1)*

For physical, symptomatic relief suggestions for massage, acupressure, and adjustment of the head plates are given in the basic analysis. Another woman asks about the cause of a white discharge from the reproductive area, often an alarming condition from fears of what it might be and an embarrassing one for what the truth might say about the woman and her lover. In this case the culprit is a chemical imbalance, often precipitated by antibiotics, that fosters an overpopulation of candida:

> *We see that this is a yeast infection. The suggestions already given are adequate for this time, particularly the goldenseal and the dong quai would provide some symptomatic relief here. There are other external applications that can be used in causing there to be some killing of the fungus and the bacteria that tends to build in this area. (4-17-93-BGC-6)*

One person discovers recent weight loss is not due to a potentially debilitating disease but to an overactive thyroid. Another learns the pain in the abdomen is from gas trapped in the intestines. A person learns that stimulating the nerve trunks in the spinal column will improve his eyesight. Another asks if there is malignancy in the body and discovers the answer is none, but there are areas of collection of dead tissue that could become *"easy sites for malignancy were this one to produce the attitudes conducive to that."* From diet to exercise, from physical environmental hazards to homeopathy, information is forthcoming on the primary disorders existing in the physical body.

Those who are acquainted with the importance of attitude, seek intuitive information to enhance self-knowledge. They expect and receive a depth of insight and understanding into issues they are cognizant of yet are finding hard to change. A young man asking, *"What is the cause of having difficulty in learning intimacy, was it something I learned this lifetime, if so where or from whom?"* discovers his problem is not with others, it is with himself:

> *Because this one believes that he is less than, he is afraid that others will discover this should this one become open and real and honest. This is a fallacy, for when this one becomes open, real, and honest, releasing the past and seeing it for what it is, beginning to respond in the present, this one will discover that he is no better than and no less than any other person. He can only be less than or better than himself. Until this one makes strides in resolving this, this one will continue to be afraid of people. (8-10-93-BGC-4)*

Learning why gives this man a place to start, a new beginning in his associations with others. A similar question concerning "overcoming the fear of being intimate with people" meets with this response:

> *Would suggest to this one that there is nothing for this one to lose when this one blends with another. We see that in order for this one to understand this, there is a need for this one to form complete thoughts. We see that because this one skims over the surface of the thinking, this one becomes very easily influenced by others and is very susceptible to the thinking of others. Would suggest that rather than this one considering this to be a fault or defect, this one learn to appreciate the ability that this one has to blend with others. In order for there to be security in this, there is a need for this one to complete this one's own thoughts so even when blending, in which there is a merging and enhancement of the self, this one knows that the self is an individual and that this one has an identity that is whole and that this cannot be lost. (10-25-92-LJF-12)*

Some questions seek peace from what haunts us. Life and death, love and loss, yearning and fulfillment. A woman asks, "What are the unresolved issues concerning my father's death when I was fifteen?"

We see that much of this one's pattern of losing is involved with this experience and the parts that this one has not understood or come to terms with. We see that it directly relates in regards to this one's feelings of security, this one's feelings of authority, this one's sense of well-being, in being safe.

Would suggest for this one to realize that this one was not abandoned purposefully. Would suggest that this one cease judging and trying to place blame upon this other one for what this one believes was lost. For it is only in reaching this point of admittance of grief that this one can begin to rebuild a sense of inner confidence, a sense of inner security, inner safety, inner authority. (1-25-94-BGC-6)

In every stage of life, through every rite of passage, what is gained from intuitive assessment is incomparable and immensely valuable to those wanting to know what they can do to ensure well-being. Whether seeking a simple answer to a complex problem or the sagacity that will initiate healing spiritually, mentally, emotionally, and physically, Intuitive Health Analyses bring to the world much more than another alternative. They bring unity. They bring cooperation. They bring answers.

They bring spiritual revolution.

Part II

Resurrection

T he first wealth is health.

Sickness is poor-spirited, and cannot serve any one;

it must husband its resources to live.

But health answers its own ends, and has to spare;

runs over, and inundates the neighborhoods and creeks

of other men's necessities.

— Ralph Waldo Emerson, 1850
American poet & essayist

G iving is the secret of a healthy life.

Not necessarily money,

but whatever a man has of

encouragement and sympathy and understanding.

— John D. Rockefeller, Jr., 1950
American capitalist & philanthropist

Rites of Passage

Much has been written about the passages in our lives, the stages of growth that come in cycles.

They are at once spiritually guided genetic patterns, universally applicable and uniquely expressed, that enable us to experience physical life fully. All great thinkers have contemplated the movement from birth to death and the relevance of what happens in between. All great Holy Scriptures of the world seek to offer spiritual guidance for how to live those years. All governments seek to bring some kind of societal order to them.

How we live our lives, what we make of ourselves in the process is eloquently described by one of my favorite creative geniuses, William Shakespeare. His exquisite depiction of how any man lives life is a testimony to the universality of our experience as human beings.

"All the world's a stage,
And all the men and women merely players.
They have their exits and their entrances;
And one man in his time plays many parts,
His acts being seven ages. At first the infant,
Mewing and puking in the nurse's arms.
And then the whining schoolboy, with his satchel,
And shining morning face, creeping like snail
Unwillingly to school. And then the lover,
Sighing like furnace, with a woeful ballad
Made to his mistress' eyebrow. Then a soldier,
Full of strange oaths, and bearded like the pard,
Jealous in honour, sudden and quick in quarrel,
Seeking the bubble reputation
Even in the cannon's mouth. And then the justice,
In fair round belly with good capon lined,
With eyes severe, and beard of formal cut,

Full of wise saws and modern instances;
And so he plays his part. The sixth age shifts
Into the lean and slippered pantaloon,
With spectacles on the nose and pouch on side,
His youthful hose well saved a world too wide
For his shrunk shank; and his big manly voice,
Turning again towards childish treble, pipes
And whistles in his sound. Last scene of all,
That ends this strange eventful history,
Is second childishness, and mere oblivion,
Sans teeth, sans eyes, sans taste, sans everything."
    – *As You Like It (1599) act 2, sc. 7, 1.139*

These seven stages of man are a perfect way to illustrate how people use Intuitive Health Analyses to live a better life at every age. You are never too old nor too young to learn and grow so you can fulfill the purpose for which you are on earth. Always be open to the spiritual advantage derived from wholistic knowledge.

A thrill fills every fiber of your being when something you have fashioned in your imagination is brought to fruition. Every artist knows the moment, so does every high school graduate, and every astronaut that leaves the planet Earth. This is the thrill of creation, bringing something into being from your own Promethean efforts.

What is universally true is that any time, anywhere, anyone draws upon the power of the mind to imagine they are manifesting the destiny of all men. The quest for a better life is inherent to human beings. The vision to include us all is a wisdom that comes as we move through the stages of man from the receptive, eager-to-learn days of infancy to the generous, willing-to-enrich nights of a lifetime well spent. Through it all good health is what is most important to any of us for with it all good things in life are better and without it even the good things are a cause for sorrow.

Here are ways, at every stage of life, people have drawn upon intuitive knowledge to ensure the health and well-being of themselves and those they love. Let these people and their histories speak for themselves.

"At first the infant"

*H*ezekiah weighed eight pounds, three ounces at birth.
He was robust and healthy. Because he was delivered by Caesarean he was not brought to me to nurse until twelve hours after his birth. By that time he'd already been given sugar water by bottle from well-meaning nurses. Being my first child I didn't yet know what that meant. At the time I just knew the last two days had not transpired as I had imagined they would, and surrendering my newborn into the care of technical professionals was part of the bargain when medical help became necessary during the delivery.

The weeks following Hezekiah's birth were challenging as I look back on it now. Although his father and I had taught and counseled countless parents over the years, we were both deficit in physical contact with newborns. I had intuitive memories of an Irish lifetime when I bore eighteen children and raised thirteen of them, but the recall centered on understandings I had made a part of myself like proper perspective and order rather than the arduous physical demands children bring. Both my husband, Daniel, and I had been in communication with the soul we called Hezekiah before his incarnation and we had spiritually prepared ourselves well, it was the newness of experience that overshadowed all else. We were in the infancy stage of the parenting experience just as our son was. So in retrospect it made sense that our first lessons would revolve around physical issues.

I had decided before Hezekiah was born that I would breastfeed for at least one year. I knew it was important for his mental and emotional growth – security, love, closeness, intelligence – as well as his physical growth. Contrary to what doctors told my mother in the 1950's, I knew mother's milk is nature's food for offspring. No matter how he tries, man will never make a replacement that is even comparable to mother's milk because no manmade formula contains the life force and antibodies present in the baby's mother's milk. Since my husband and I were not planning to subject our son to being given small doses of viruses – those causing polio, pertussus, diphtheria, tetanus, it's called immunization in medical circles – passing on my immunity was paramount for our son's protection.

So we nursed what seemed like constantly. It moved in three hour cycles throughout the day. Hezekiah would nurse for at least twenty minutes per breast. At night he would nurse between 10 and 11 o'clock, then awaken around 2 or 3, and again at 6 or 7 to start a new day. I tried to nap with him but after several weeks my lack of deep sleep was wearing on me. And most alarming, Hezekiah was slow in gaining weight.

He had lost the usual three or so ounces in the week following his birth. But in the four weeks following he had failed to regain back to his birth weight. At weekly visits with the doctor who delivered him we asked about this, showing increasing concern. The doctor was not at all alarmed for Kie was gaining and said if he didn't gain more in the next couple weeks we might need to supplement his diet with formula.

Daniel and I talked about the possibility of needing to supplement Kie's nourishment with the vitamin concoctions commonly sold. We considered fresh cow's milk, available from the College of Metaphysics' animal husbandry department, but ruled against it because of possible bacteria and the nutrients pasteurizing would kill.

My major concern was that Hezekiah might stop nursing if we started him on a bottle. I had read from more than one source that babies easily switch from breast to bottle because the bottle is more forthcoming and takes less effort. I also knew Hezekiah's skull and brain development needed the extra exertion that he was making by sucking at breast. And I wanted to be able to give my son what he needed. We'd done so well while he was in the womb that I didn't understand why we seemed to be having trouble now. So we were also dealing with a new mother's fragile ego and hormone influenced emotions.

The most obvious course of action for Daniel and me was what we knew and trusted the most, an Intuitive Health Analysis. As a third opinion, after my husband's and my own, we knew the analysis would clear the air of any misconceptions we had, offer an objective point of view, and lend insights into the experience of a six-week-old human being. It met our expectations and more.

The analysis began, as always, with a report on Hezekiah's mental system. What was described verified the knowledge we had gained over the years in our research indicating an infant's completely receptive nature of consciousness:

> *We see that this one is very sensitive to the environment. We see that there is a tendency for this one to be drawn to stimuli that are strong and we see that therefore this one's attention is continually pulled from one stimulus to another. We see that there is the need for this one to focus upon particular stimuli that are appealing to this one. Would suggest that there be direction given to this one in order for this one to begin to choose the stimuli that this one wants to absorb.*

Daniel and I were providing constant care. The only time Hezekiah lay in his bassinet unattended was when he was sleeping and oftentimes he was held by one of us then. We talked and sang to him, cradled and walked him sometimes hours into the night.

I had been somewhat of a hermit these weeks, regaining strength from the surgery and adjusting to the new element of our family. Neither Kie nor I had made too many appearances outside our living quarters. Our community was a busy one, living on the College of Metaphysics campus with other faculty members and students, so it was easy to begin imagining how he could receive more and varied stimuli just by incorporating more people into his daily life. By the analysis we knew it was time for more varied contact.

We also became more aware of the stimulus in Hezekiah's environment. What to us might be the chance to watch a late movie on television was for Kie a series of sounds, sometimes filled with ominous musical tones and alarming noises of crises, that when I realized it I saw no good reason to subject my son to it. Or trying to get him interested in stroking a stuffed animal so he'd stop crying when what he needed was sensory relief in the form of another diaper change. Or the tendency to have background music playing while talking to him. We could do better than giving Hezekiah two sensory inputs at the same time by being more sensitive to the environment ourselves.

> *We see that within the emotional system that this one is also sensitive. We see that once again there are many different stimuli that this one is subject to. Sounds. Emotions of other people.*

Different temperatures. We see that this one is especially sensitive
to sound and variations in sound. We see that it would benefit this
one to receive soothing sounds, soothing textures.

We knew all children up to the age of seven are subject to the emotions of those in the environment, and for this reason Daniel and I kept our own focus on the love and care of our newborn. Years of concentration exercises were definitely being applied during those early days. As we created more and more ways to soothe Kie, we found they also helped soothe us.

The information on the physical system was equally enlightening. It introduced me to the entire concept of how the newborn human needs nine more months in order to be able to sustain itself apart from the mother, but because of the evolutionary changes in the human species, for instance the upright stance and the size of the brain and skull, birth must transpire when the fetus is still underdeveloped in many ways. Nine months enables the respiratory system to be sufficiently developed to sustain life, but it does not give sufficient time for the nervous system and digestive system to be adequately developed. This happens after physical birth and is the reason so many newborns struggle with the radical change that birth brings in assimilating food. Because it is not understood, it is seen as a disease and even given a name, colic, when in reality it is a natural evolvement of the growing body. Kie's reading described this very well:

We see that within the physical system there is a great degree of
sensitivity in the nervous system, the digestive system, and as a
result the eliminatory system. We see that there are toxins that are
attempting to be released from the intestines and the digestive tract.
We see that these also release themselves through the skin. Would
suggest that it would benefit this one to be touched on the skin in a
stroking fashion. This would aid to some extent in causing the
release of the toxins. We see that the intake of small amounts of
water would benefit this one. We see that small amounts of rice
water would be beneficial. We see that gentle massage of the bottom
of the feet would be beneficial.

One of the students at the College was a certified massage therapist and one of her passions was infant massage. She generously offered to teach me the series of movements that had been proven to benefit newborns. I began massaging him at least once a day and I could see progress in how well he kept his food down and how his legs were relaxing more, extending, and fists beginning to open. Massage times became special times of spiritual rapport for Hezekiah and me. I knew I was helping his soul to adjust to the limits of his new physical body.

> *We see that there are particular sounds that could be used that would be soothing to this one. We see that prior to or while this one is receiving nutrition that this could provide a kind of focusing for this one. We see that small amounts of exposure to sunlight would benefit this one. This would be for short periods of time. This is all.*

Then came the big questions, the stimulus for us to request Hezekiah's first Intuitive Health Analysis. My husband asked, "This entity (Hezekiah) is gaining weight slowly or not at all for the last couple of weeks, and has not regained his original birth weight. What is the cause of this and any suggestions?" The answer was clear, relieving any fear of a more complicated problem and affirming what we had concluded:

> *We see that this one has difficulty assimilating nutrients. We see that a lower sugar content in the nutrition that this one is receiving would aid.*

> Question: This entity is being breastfed is there anything the mother can do then to lower the sugar content?
> *Eliminate refined sugar and use molasses; molasses would be the best sweetener. The elimination of chocolate would be recommended also.*

> Q: Is the child receiving enough nutrition from the mother's milk?
> *We see that the kind of nutrition is adequate, we see that the quantity is somewhat deficient. We see that drinking a small amount of rice water would aid in this one being able to digest the nutrition to a better extent.*

> Q: Is this one receiving adequate liquid in the breast milk, particularly the hindmilk that is rich in fat?
> *No.*

Q: Any suggestions for the one of the mother in having more liquid? Is this one sucking properly, positioned at the breast properly?
Would suggest to the one of the mother to drink water throughout the day. It would be recommended that this one drink small amounts of water every hour throughout the day....

Q: Would supplementary formula in addition to breast milk give assistance in weight gain?
We see that this could provide some benefit. We see that goat's milk would also provide some benefit...

Q: Is the digestive system capable of assimilating and using formula milk without constipation?
We see that there would be some constipation. We see that plain water used alternatively would aid... (3-10-95-LJC-8)

The analysis told us what we needed to know. We began supplementing Hezekiah's diet that evening. For such a small physical change it held profound meaning for me. It was a ritual experience, highly emotional, a giving of my son to his father in a way I had not been able to because the birth was high-tech rather than natural. At his birth a doctor we had just met cut the umbilical cord tying mother and son and some nurse we didn't know handed our newborn to my husband. Now weeks later the sense of family that had been interrupted in a bright, sterile hospital room was at last consummated in the comforting warmth of our bedroom. Mother, father, child. We could relish the ritual that every set of parents has known letting it sink into our consciousness and transform its magic. For all the trials of the learning attached to it, that moment of first offering Hezekiah a bottle is a memory I will always cherish for how it brought us together as a family.

The analysis had confirmed that we would be doing the right thing to give Kie manmade infant formula, that it would not be harmful, and could be soothing to him. I put out extra effort to keep nursing and did so until Kie came down with the flu following a holiday visit at his Grandad's. For a week Hezekiah was reduced to mostly mouth breathing which made him resistant to breastfeeding and eager for the ease of a bottle. From that time on he preferred bottle to breast and fairly quickly he was weaned, a couple weeks shy of the year I had set. But for months we continued to nurse and I will always be glad of the choice I made in that regard.

Bottlefeeding gave Daniel a chance for the bonding that had been Hezekiah's and mine. The pride and sheer pleasure Dan derived from these mealtimes with Kie was obvious. I found myself many times very thankful that everything had unfolded as it did.

Daniel would feed Hezekiah from a bottle, I would breastfeed. I thought this would help Kie continue to nurse, and it worked. He also began to associate certain kinds of food with Dad and certain kinds with Mama. It eased my schedule tremendously giving me freedom to sleep a bit more since Dan was now able to supply one of the middle of the night feedings.

The report also gave us insights that at least helped us to understand our newborn's experience. As every parent knows, we were learning to interpret Hezekiah's language which in the first months consisted of mostly crying. I wanted to know if there were any reasons for him crying other than those Dan and I had already identified: from hunger, wet diapers, and digestive pain.

We see that these are the primary causes. We see that there are also times when this one desires to stretch the limbs or to exercise the limbs and does not know how. We see that the ones of the parents could aid by offering gentle resistance to this one's legs in particular for this one to push against.

I also wanted to know what we could do to help Hezekiah adjust to his new body, to make it more comfortable. His constant battle with gas caused him to lose much of the milk he took in, often woke him from sleep, and was definitely controlling all our lives. Most importantly I wanted to be sure that he was fully formed and growing properly. The report allayed any fear in this regard and gave some helpful suggestions:

Question: Is there any other reason other than gas or being too full for this one spitting up?
We see that this one is still in the process of learning how to adequately assimilate the nutrition to draw what is needed by the body and to eliminate the rest. We see that this is a natural process of elimination.

Q: Is this one on the way to gaining this ability to digest?
To some extent. We see that touching the skin would accelerate this.

Q: Are digestive discomforts, that is gas, due to newness and adjustment to the body?

We see for the most part this is a natural process of adjustment. We do see that reducing the refined sugar content in the mother's diet would aid. We see that this is also because of the sensitivity to the environment, many different stimuli that capture this one's attention. And oftentimes this one does not have the full attention on digestion when the food is in the system. Therefore, aiding this one to give the full attention to the digestion rather than being distracted by other stimuli would benefit.

Once I knew Hezekiah was adjusting well, I felt freer to examine how and why the difficulty with adequate nourishment from breastfeeding had happened to us. Beyond what the analysis told us about our son, I could now focus on what it told me about *me*. The first thing I learned was the problem I had with dehydration in my body was severe enough to interfere with my capacity to breastfeed. Looking back I remember that just about every Intuitive Health Analysis I had ever received had suggested I drink more water or fluids. Having been on the road day in and day out for years during my mid-20's to latter 30's I had become used to drinking minimal amounts so I wouldn't have to waste time stopping to relieve myself. When I did drink it was not water, it was tea or coffee or soda all notorious for their diuretic effects.

Now I was confronted with my own neglect. I knew I had been dehydrated the final twelve hours of labor. Once I left the birthing center and my midwife's care and entered into the hospital and medical care I was hooked to machines and not allowed any liquids although I repeatedly asked for them. Before going to surgery I was completely dry and I knew it. What I didn't know was the effect this would have on nursing. Now it seems quite obvious that breast milk is made of fluids in mom's body, but at the time other concerns were more pressing so this awareness came later.

Even after giving birth, it was hours before I was allowed to drink and a day before I was given food to eat. On top of this add the drugs that were used during surgery. My system was way out of balance.

Once I got home I tried to drink more but as Kie's reading said I still wasn't drinking enough. Drinking meant releasing what is no longer needed and my bladder was weak from the pregnancy and surgery plus I wasn't moving real fast yet. So I drank but I didn't drink as much as I needed. At the time this seemed like reasons rather than excuses. However, there was no denying that my failure to drink enough fluids directly affected my capacity to nurse.

Even on formula Kie still took the full nine months to adjust to life outside the womb. The Intuitive Health Analysis was a necessary part of our understanding of our newborn and our own peace of mind.

We have known for years that what parents can learn during an Intuitive Health Analysis on their child is phenomenal. It is easily a teaching tool, a personal textbook for better parenting, a guide for wholistic health care not only for the child but the parents as well. The questions it answers are alone worth the money invested, and what parent will not pay any price to ensure his child's good health? Health analyses point the way to health and well-being, responding to what is needed now and why. For first time parents this knowledge is invaluable. For parents with problems it is a household peacemaker. For parents with difficult health care choices to make it offers a different perspective that can make those choices easier to understand. And what parent has not wondered what's going on in the mind of their six-month-old?– An Intuitive Health Analysis will tell you.

I have worked with parents who were concerned that their quarreling was affecting their children. Parents have asked about medications, therapies, diet, sports activities. They have asked about sibling rivalries, friends, peer pressure, and the development of social skills. Parents have been concerned about intellectual development, learning abilities, and creative stimulus. In every case, Intuitive Health Analyses report the truth that exists. They also give suggestions for parents and child to foster growth and maturity of the child's full potential.

Now Daniel and I are benefiting from the same service we have offered others for two decades. We hope to multiply the goodwill by contributing what we learn about parenting the soul. Toward this end, every six months we request an Intuitive Health Analysis on our son. We intend to do so until he reaches the age of seven or so when he will be old enough to understand and request intuitive reports himself. Eventually these analyses, what they convey and how they are effectively applied in our lives, will be the subject of a book for parents.

We know each Intuitive Health Analysis we request on Hezekiah is a gauge of the spiritual guidance we are providing him through example and through instruction. The analyses are an incomparable educational source for Hezekiah's stages of learning and his *capacity* to learn. They are a check-up on physical development and nourishment. They are a continuing source of insight helping us to be the best parents we can be.

I keep thinking what a different experience souls in young bodies will have when all parents want to use intuitively-accessed information to help their child mature, not only physically but spiritually. The number of drug dependent kids will decrease, not street drugs but medically sanctioned drugs, the labeling of children as difficult, impaired, or deficient will become passe, and parents will begin assuming responsibility for the offspring they bring into the world. Responsible parents raise their children giving time, love, and attention to them instead of passing them to a nanny or daycare owner to hopefully supply what they are not. Responsible parents teach their children standards and the discipline to meet them instead of dumping uncivilized illiterates on underpaid teachers at governmentally-run schools. Responsible parents spiritually guide their children instead of leaving them to their own devices without any moral compass. Responsible parents do not blame others for their own failing, they look to see what they can do in the best interest of their child and *they do it.*

Intuitive Health Analyses make that work a lot easier. They tell as much about the parents as they do about the child being observed and analyzed. In that way, it is a report on three people instead of just one; intuitive insight into the health of the family itself. Every family can grow from such wisdom.

"And then the whining schoolboy"

"**W**hen the eyes, nose and throat specialist started talking about putting tubes in my son's ears, I decided before I allowed that to happen I would get a health reading."

Her son Beau was almost four and had already received the "antibiotic treatment and everything else that was going on at that time" in an effort to cure her son's recurring ear infections. The thought of her son's eardrum being burst was just a bit too radical for her. It was time to do something else.

"Because of the environment I grew up in – with a father who was a pharmacist who spoke with people all the time about health – early on I realized that doctors weren't gods. They are human and they make mistakes, they misprescribe. This plus experiences I had growing up where something was undiagnosed or undiagnosable kept me open to alternatives.

"At the age of 26 I had my first health analysis because I had some symptoms that looked like hypoglycemia and I didn't want to go through the glucose tolerance test. My friend Michael Clark told me to give it a try, the health analyses are one of their most valuable tools. And I said okay I'll give it a try. I'll do that before I go do a glucose test. These symptoms I was having were pretty severe. I would have moments of being paranoid, anxious. My mind would race and I would shake uncontrollably. It was interfering with my work and therefore my business.

"The first part in the reading talked about what was going on in the mental system which was the *"lack of self love"*. When it got into the physical there was hypoglycemia, borderline diabetes, and at that point it recommended chiropractic care. Everything that was related in that analysis hit home with me and so I didn't really want to like that analysis. I didn't want to believe it was any good so I went to a chiropractor, my mother's, to x-ray my spine. All the vertebrae that were in that report were confirmed by the x-ray. At that point I went out and got my book on learning to love myself.

So in June, 1987, she requested the first Intuitive Health Analysis for Beau. "The reason I got the reading was that he complained about his stomach hurting, headaches, and also the earaches. We found out about those and a lot more."

We see that within the mental system there is being formed an idea of stubbornness which this one is using in order to establish this one's own importance. We see that in many ways that this one is attempting to build an identity of the self which is separate from those around the self but because there is not the consistency in this one's environment this one becomes either temperamental or very withdrawn and very secretive.

We see that there is a need for this one to be stimulated particularly in areas of concentration but also in areas which would stimulate this one's imagination. We see that reading stories that would require this one visualizing and imaging would be of benefit to this one. We see also that those things which would require combinations of color, shape and texture would be of benefit in stimulating the imagination as well.

We see that in many ways this one becomes somewhat anxious when there is the restlessness being expressed by others around the self because this one immediately looks to the self as wanting to establish a continuity or a consistency or an ease in what this one sees as a disease or an imbalance or restlessness. We see that when this occurs this one becomes somewhat confused and begins to try and identify with the restlessness as opposed to identifying with what it is that could be used or learned.

We see that this one is very manipulative in nature and very creative in the way that this one uses manipulation but loses some sight of the self when it backfires and this one finds the self separated from those that this one has depended upon. We see that in many ways those around the self view themselves in a harsh and critical manner and this is reflected in the communication and in the attitudes that are held which does promote the need on this one's part to fulfill those desires. We see this to be affecting the mental and emotional systems.

We see within the area of the physical system that there are not major disorders. We see that there is some sluggishness within the colon area particularly and that because of this there is not the absorbing of the nutrients from the substances that are taken into the system. We see that through the use of massage to the abdomen area this would aid in stimulating motion within the colon area and would also stimulate some absorption processing of the food substances. We see that this one is quite capable of handling many varieties of food substances but is defining or beginning to establish a pattern that limits the willingness to take in food substances. Would suggest that this has to do with the reflection of the attitudes of those around the self as to what is pleasant and what is unpleasant.

We see that within the area of the respiratory system there is congestion and that this is due to indecision. We see that the inhalation of the vapors of steam combined with eucalyptus and menthol would provide some relief to this area.

We do see that there is an imbalance in the fluid levels within the inner ear area that does produce some difficulty in the maintaining of balance and coordination for this one. Would suggest that there be a cleansing of this area. Would suggest also that pressure be applied in the form of acupressure around the ears and the base of the skull. We see that there is a slight misalignment in the second and fourth cervical, the third and fifth thoracic. Would suggest chiropractic attention in this. This is all. (6-2-87-GBM-a)

"It had dawned on me to go to the chiropractor right around the time that the analysis came in. The earache problem happened to him at eight months. I had him adjusted (by a chiropractor) and everything was fine up until this time. Once I heard the analysis I thought of course! However, at that point for me, everything had to do with the mental and the emotional dynamics. When the ears became a problem to the extent that they wanted to do something like tubes in his ears, that's when I thought to have an analysis done for Beau to find out what was going on in the mental and emotional.

"I got what I was looking for.

"The colon problems described in the analysis addressed Beau's constipation and also let us know he wasn't absorbing the nutrients from the substances that were taken into the system. *'We see that this one is quite capable of handling many varieties of food substance but is defining or beginning to establish a pattern that limits the willingness to take in food substances.'* Beau had always been real open to any type of food that I gave him. The only thing that he would not eat was sushi. He would eat anything.

"Bob (Terri's husband) and I had different experiences growing up. He had opinions about children and food substances, what they could and could not take and he believed that children could only take sweet or salty. He began to cook for Beau – French fries and fish sticks. I was totally against it. However, he was the house-husband so to speak and I was the working person. So he did the majority of the cooking at that time and I did not. I was too busy rushing about. So I believe that that also had something to do with the colon area. But what's funny is that Bob's health analysis revealed that he had the same thing with the colon, my analysis had the same thing with the colon.

"All three of us had respiratory problems. And at that time we also took the carpets that were in our house out and old duct work that was in the A/C and they were cleaned. Beau's analysis was like a family health analysis, because he was at that age such a direct reflection of my husband and me.

"My life was crazy at that time. I was running a salon with six hair dressers and pretty manipulative in my own way. Pretty temperamental in my own ways as well. In a lot of ways, this analysis is such a blend of what Bob and I were going through. In my health analysis that was at the very same time, I had a lot of impatience and intolerance. I wasn't communicating well or wasn't communicating at all. Nor was I consistent in action progressively. With Bob's at that point, just speaking off the top of my head, he was anxious most of the time. I don't think he even knew. There was a lot of harshness that both of us — I would say Beau was around a lot of harshness, a lot of criticalness, manipulativeness, restrictiveness with both parents not being able to express emotionally. I think at that point I was living life the way I thought that I was supposed to and real frustrated with it — having a certain amount of knowledge about things but not being able to put it together. In wanting to help but not knowing how to help."

In this first analysis, the conductor asked on her behalf if there were further suggestions for the mother. The answer was just what Terri needed to hear.

Would suggest that there is a racing in this one's thoughts when there is communication with this one. We see that because of that there is inconsistency in the expectations and inconsistency on the willingness to follow through. Because of this there is insecurity that is fostered in this one by the ones around the self. Therefore, it is when there will be the consistency, the full attention when there is communication and the willingness to follow through upon what is seen to be correct which would aid both of these ones. This is all. (6-2-87-GBM-a)

"I was racing in my thoughts. What I started to do differently at that point was — when I talked with Beau — I would kneel down and look at him in the eye. I would give him my attention when he spoke to me and when I spoke to him. At this suggestion, I began to make an effort to do so. At first I believe it was surprising to him. It would startle him when I would get down like that and just kind of focus all of my attention on him. During that time period he would kind of stutter. When he would talk he would say 'ummmm,' more thinking about what he wanted to say than saying it. He would repeat the same sentence over and over, and then he would finally get it out. When I would kneel down and be eye-to-eye with him, if he started that I'd say 'Beau I want you to slow down for a second and I want you to think about what you want to say and then say it.' And he would. By me slowing down and giving him my attention Beau could do the same.

"This analysis really brought to my attention that when I asked Beau to do something or started to direct his attention to do something, that I needed to stay with him on it until it was completed. Mean what I say and just stay with it.

"One of the things that I was concerned about was that Beau would withdraw and he would be secretive. And I knew when he would do that but I wasn't sure what that was all about and the analysis brought up that subject."

*K*nowing first hand what an Intuitive Health Analysis gives the parent, Terri used these analyses as a check-up or in the case of problems. By the time Beau was 6 years he knew about the intuitive reports and was listening to them because he wanted to know what was happening to him.

The next report was perhaps the most enigmatic of all his analyses for Terri, particularly with the physical difficulties. She would find much of what was revealed here was a description of who her son was becoming and the impact his environment was having on his sense of self-worth. At the time of this report Beau was six and well into kindergarten.

> *This one has a very firm image of the self. We see that this one has adopted a devil-may-care attitude which this one professes and puts out to other individuals. We see that this makes this one appear as happy-go-lucky and as being able to handle anything that is thrown his way. However, underneath this facade is the actuality of what this one lives in his own thinking. And we see that in this regard this one does not want to take things seriously but does. This one wants to be able to handle things but feels inadequate and we see that this one does not like to consider these things for he sees it as weakness and this one disdains weakness. We see that there is almost a type of self hate because of this and we see that there is great difficulty in this one refusing to admit who this one is, where this one has come from, and where this one wants to go.*

"You notice how it says, *'underneath this facade is the actuality of what this one lives in his own thinking.'* He wants *'to be able to handle things but feels inadequate.'* It was a bit disconcerting until we discovered what it was all about. One day his teacher says, 'Terri, he's got this whole book memorized. He doesn't read it.' She snapped when he held the book upside down reading. He wasn't reading, he was memorizing. Beau would *memorize* books. He tested on a fourth grade level for environmental and below his age group for reading and writing and math. So we got into this. They (school officials) began pressuring me to get Beau tested, 'there is something not right with him', 'he has a learning disability'."

> *Would suggest that this one cease causing there to be such great strain upon the self by thinking in the ways that have been described and begin to become more real and more honest in terms of who this one is and who this one wants to become.*

It was obvious Beau couldn't continue to fake it, and his efforts to do so were affecting not only his relationships with others but who he believed himself to be.

> *Would suggest that this one has many assets for the self but they are not often used because of the ways that this one has filled the mind*

with creations of this facade that has been described. Would suggest that this one become much more invested in being able to recognize who this one is and what this one's skills, talents and abilities are and put them to use in the life. This would lead to a much more productive existence and a much happier one for this one as well.

"We started reading books. Just reading, just to relax. Actually at that point the reading wasn't relaxing to him. Probably because it was a tense situation for him. We started doing tapes like the healing waterfall and guided imagery tapes which even today if he's not feeling his best he'll listen to those tapes. Or he'll listen to them at night to go to sleep.

We see the emotions for the most part to be ignored. We see that this one has a particular set emotional pattern that this one allows the self to indulge in and this one, although he experiences other emotions, does not admit them. Therefore, these are suppressed and we see that they do cause difficulties in the body at times.

"A lot is ignored in the emotions. Well Beau had a great pattern going for that with Bob because Bob at that point only had one way. I don't think he was aware of emotions or what they were. And of course, I was just perfect with everything."

Would suggest that this one become more honest with the emotions as well and begin to realize that admitting what exists is not have to admit weakness. It is not a matter of whether this one is weak or strong. It is a matter of this one's willingness to admit what exists and to face facts and to learn how to use facts productively. Would suggest that this is part of the ability of a reasoner and that as long as this one is not doing this, this one is not reasoning but is relying very heavily upon habitual, compulsive patterns and emotional reactions. In this way this one is being weak, being what this one most does not want.

"Then we get into the physical. This is the analysis that I got that confused me. I really didn't understand and this is one of the reasons I point out to parents if there is information on a report you don't understand talk to an alternative health care practitioner. Ask them what they know. And if they don't know it find somebody else who does know it.

We see within the physical body that there is some difficulty in the heart and circulatory system. We see that there is tendency toward arrhythmia in the heart. Would suggest that this one learn how to relax, not only physically but mentally and emotionally as well. We see that there is a need for more blood to be pumped through the circulatory system. Would suggest exercise which would cause a beating of the heart more regularly. This would not be taxing exercise, but it could be in the line of sports. We see that within the digestive system that there is some difficulty in the liver. There is only about two thirds of this area that is functioning. Part of this is due to chemical residue. Would suggest that this one eliminate any type of substance which does not have a nutritional value.

Q: Would this produce stomach pains?
We see that those are related. However, we see the stomach pains to be more directly associated with light ulcerations which are occurring in the stomach area. Would suggest more bland foods. Would suggest more dairy products, particularly milk, in the diet.

Q: What would be causing the ulcerations?
We see that this is a type of — the type of self-hatred that has been described, this is where it manifests. It is in worry that this one is going to be caught.

Continue.

We see that there is some difficulty in the action of the colon as well. We see that the dairy products that have been given would aid and more water in this one's diet would aid. We see that this is a type of spastic action which is inconsistent and is not conducive to evacuation of waste material on a regular basis. We see that because of the liver and the colon and even the difficulties in the stomach that there is a tendency toward toxicity in this body and this reacts in a variety of ways. It reacts through the respiratory system in attempting to rid itself of toxins and in regards to the skin glands and trying to rid itself of waste, to a certain extent the kidneys. The addition of water will at least give a vehicle for the toxins to be removed from the body. We see that these toxins for the most part are made up of waste materials that have not gained exit from the body any other way or in the normal channels which would be primarily through the colon and the urethra. This is all.... (10-3-89-BGO)

"I could readily understand *'there is some difficulty in the heart and circulatory'* and it goes on with arrhythmia in the heart and that he needed to learn how to relax. Well you know when you are putting on a facade at school that you can read when you can't, you know something is wrong with you but you don't know what it is. So from there it talks about the blood being pumped through the circulatory system and the heart beating more regularly, no taxing exercise but something in the line of sports. He began martial arts for the mental discipline as much as for the exercise.

"Now here's where it gets interesting, in the digestive system there is some difficulty in the liver. Well when I got that I kind of went, 'Huh? what could be going on with his liver?' And then from there it says that part of this is due to chemical residue. He was having stomach pains at that time period which the reading described as light ulcerations, manifestations of *'the type of self-hatred that has been described, this is where it manifests and is in a worry that this one is going to be caught.'* Here Beau was, he was fearing he was going to be found out. We could help him change that. Beau also had little bitty bumps on his skin, a manifestation of the body attempting to rid itself through the skin glands of waste. We could also help cleanse his body.

"Among the questions we asked if there were suggestions for Bob and me as parents:

> *Would suggest that these ones become much more invested in discovering who this one is, in stimulating this one to think and encouraging the expression of his ideas rather than attempting to mold this one in a certain way which is not this one's way, which is not in alignment with what this one thinks. We see that in the ways that these ones express many times there is the judgmentalness of right or wrong which this one has learned to take into the self and misuse in the ways that have already been described. Would suggest that rather than right or wrong, punishment or reward, this one be taught responsibility. This is all.*

"I do believe at that point we were telling Beau who he was supposed to be, what he was supposed to be, even though he was supposed to be special.

He's supposed to be special in a certain way. Yeah and we were definitely into what's right, wrong, punishment, reward, and responsibility. Even now years later I can think right off the top of my head, of an example of the punishment or reward. He was biting kids at school and at that age children don't usually do that. I bribed him with M&Ms. It worked. And in another year, Beau's over indulgence in soda pop and candy, the enormous amounts of sugar he consumed, would be a health concern revealed in another analysis."

The prospect that Beau might have a learning disability preyed in the back of Terri's mind.

"I didn't get all the testing that the kindergarten teacher wanted me to get done because it would have cost me anywhere from $10,000 to $20,000. At least that was the estimate I had from parents who had done this with their children. I could have had it done for $800 but what they put children through to do that, I didn't want to put that on Beau. I talked with different people, principals, people in the educational system. I talked to a pediatrician and at that point it was decided that I would wait until Beau had gone through first grade to make a decision on what I was going to do with him.

"We came to the summer of '91, Beau had completed first grade. I went to his first grade teacher and I said, 'Miss, I want to ask you something. How do you feel Beau is as a student? Do you feel like he has learning disabilities?' 'Terri, I strongly suspect Beau's dyslexic.' She says, 'I went to my mother who is also a teacher of many years beyond mine and I told her about Beau and what my mother told me is teach him different.'

"Well I had learned this with Beau already when the kindergarten teacher couldn't teach him how to subtract and get the whole concept of subtraction, I took ten teddy bears out and put them on his bed and said, 'There's ten teddy bears. You know, you've got five fingers here and five fingers here, that makes ten fingers. Now if I take two teddy bears away, how many teddy bears are left.' He said, 'eight'. I said, 'That's subtraction Beau.' Well we're still trying to wean him off his fingers but it worked. So what she said made sense to me. However, I wanted to go ahead and get a current Intuitive Health Analysis to find out if there were problems or learning disabilities. It was my first question: 'Do you find any learning disabilities with the visual perception?'

> *We see that the difficulty with the visual perception is related to the misalignment in the skull plates and also to some extent the atlas and axis. We do see that this does cause there to be difficulty in this one receiving clearly through this system. We do not see this to be a learning disability, however.*

> Q: Any suggestions for aiding this one?
> *Chiropractic correction would aid in terms of the physical difficulty. Would suggest that this one practice exercises which would strengthen this one's ability to concentrate and to understand what the attention is and how to direct and use the attention by giving the attention along with the use of the eyesight. (7-9-91-LJF)*

We took off across the United States and had his skull plates realigned.

"I had started transcribing Beau's analyses prior to this so I knew prior analyses had noted a chemical residue and skull plate misalignments. I took him to Jerry Coach, a chiropractor in Houston. I did not give him the information on the intuitive reports, I just asked him to examine Beau and tell me what he saw, what he thought was going on with him. Jerry Coach used kinesiology to detect the misalignment of Beau's skull plates, plates that were putting pressure on the optic nerve which was what the intuitive analysis said. He quoted me a price of about $1,200 a month to work with Beau for an extended period of time.

"That's when I went to Minneapolis to consult with Lucille, a health care professional and friend. I told Lucille that my gut feeling was that Beau didn't need that. She agreed and we went from there to a nutritionist. I let her do her thing with him and she said that his liver wasn't fully functioning because of a chemical residue which was on the analysis prior to the current one. The first question that she asked us was "Do you give him antihistamines?" And what mother this day and age who doesn't know better doesn't give their child antihistamines. It's just over-the-counter – got a runny nose, take this. Don't worry about the colon or whatever else that is associated to it. So at that point she went further to tell us that the reason there was such an increase in prostate cancer was the use of over-the-counter antihistamines. I was as guilty as the next mother for wanting a quick relief, but no more. I'd find other solutions.

"Coming back from Minneapolis, Beau started to read the signs on the side of the road and license plates and it was the first time he ever really read. That was the first summer he ever rode a bike."

Terri got the peace of mind that comes from having your questions answered and even more so from receiving suggestions of productive lines of action. As she had come to expect she also found a detailed description of what was going on in her child's mind.

We see within this one there is a great deal of secrecy that this one practices. We see that there is a particular image this one has created and does go to great lengths to maintain. We see therefore when this one does experience thoughts or perceptions or attitudes that are not in alignment with this image this one is creating, this one does attempt to hide these from others.

We see that in the process of hiding these from others this one has also developed a kind of insecurity in that this one does hide from the self the awareness of what this one's thoughts truly are. Would suggest to this one that in order for this one to be at ease with the self that there is a need for this one to practice honesty. Would suggest that this one practice some form of concentration in which this one is listening to this one's own thoughts.

Would suggest as well that this one practice communicating this one's thoughts in verbal form. Would suggest that counseling could be beneficial. Would suggest that writing could be beneficial. Would suggest that even this one using another person to speak this one's thoughts to, (someone) this one does trust could be beneficial. This type of communication needs to be very direct and straightforward in which this one is not trying to put an impression or reveal only certain thoughts but where the goal is for this one to cause there to be an external expression of the thoughts that this one does have. We see this would aid this one in then determining which thoughts this one wants to practice, which thoughts this one wants to change, which thoughts are being productive, and which thoughts are being destructive. Would suggest that this one need not fear being found out, as this one sees it, because it is only this one's own self that is trying to hide.

We see that within the emotional system there is secrecy here as well. We do see this one does have difficulty in understanding emotion, for we do see when this one does feel any type of emotion, particularly those that are stimulated from a source that this one is not aware of, that this one does interpret this as wrong. Would suggest to this one that in order for this one to have the full use of this one's power, there is a need for this one to understand the use of emotion.

Would suggest to this one this does not mean that this one must be out of control. Would suggest to this one this is not a fault on this one's part but this is a part of this one's mind and a part of this one's self. Through the directed use of this one's imagination this one could cause the expression of emotion. Would suggest to this one that this be approached as a kind of experimentation and a kind of practice and that this one formulate a goal and purpose for this based on this one discovering the power that this one does have.

We see within the physical body there is difficulty in the spleen, the kidneys, liver and gall bladder. We do see that there is not a full functioning of the spleen and that there is a difficulty within the area of the liver in processing and removing toxins from the body. We see that there is a kind of toxic condition that is occurring and we see that this does have other effects. We see that there are times when this one does experience headaches. We see that there are times when this one does experience a great sluggishness in this one's energy. Would suggest that in order for this to be corrected there would need to be changes within the mental attitudes but particularly it would be in regards to this one causing the expression of this one's emotion that this would release the energy that is available for this one's use. Would suggest that for a period of time that this one use a kind of cleansing fast in which this one drinks water and fruit juices. We see that this could be done for a period of a day. Would suggest that this one could also consult some type of nutritional expert for guidance in using other types of fasts for longer periods of time that would provide cleansing for the body. We do see that without supervision this would not be recommended for a long period of time. Would suggest the intake of warm lemon water upon arising. Would suggest the intake of small amounts of olive oil be taken in this one ingesting this pure rather than used in cooking. We see that there is a need for ginseng.

We do see that there is some difficulty within the reproductive system. We see that there is a slight enlargement in the prostate and that at times there is also irritation in the urethra. Would suggest that this one take in more water in the diet, particularly when this one is eating foods that are highly acidic. Would suggest cranberry juice and pineapple juice be taken in .

We see that there is misalignment in the skull plates. We see that this does produce a kind of pressure within the area of the head. We see that this does at times interfere with the visual system. Would suggest that these be corrected. Would suggest the use of acupressure around the area of the eyes and the back of the neck. We see that there is misalignment in the atlas, axis, third cervical, fourth cervical, ninth and tenth thoracic. We see that there is also a slight scoliosis in the lower area of the spine. We see that this in itself does not produce a difficulty but that when this one does sit putting the weight unevenly, or does stand putting the weight unevenly, that the spine does not support the body properly and then this throws the rest of the spine out of alignment. Would suggest therefore that this one practice correcting the posture. We see that hatha yoga exercises would aid in strengthening the muscles and building flexibility within the area of the spine.

We see that there is a need for more fresh vegetables in the diet, particularly green leafy vegetables, celery. We see that there is a need for more fiber. Would suggest to this one that vegetables be eaten that are raw, that this one eat apples and other foods that are crunchy. This would provide stimulus for the digestion as well as exercise for the teeth and gums for we do see that there is a kind of build up of fluid within the area of the gums and that this area does need stimulation. Vitamin C would also help within this area. This is all... (7-9-91-LJF)

"There was a lot that was going on around him at this point. Just before this analysis, there was a situation in our marriage that since we didn't have full and complete communication we had started living totally different lives and I was like doing the silent rebellion dance. One thing led to another and I was real close to having an affair. Bob was in his own way not knowing and he was also involved with massage therapy at the time. I took a trip to Mexico with a girlfriend partly to get away from everything and try to make some decisions. When I was there I read the book *Going in Circles: Our Search for a Satisfying Relationship* and I made some decisions to make the relationship work and stay committed to it.

"Bob and I went to a marriage counselor who wanted us to spend $800 to $1,000 in therapy a month and Bob and I agreed *that* was enough to cause a divorce. So we started requesting past life profiles and past life crossings every three to four months for insight and to help us understand each other. If we needed to, we would go to a Unity church minister and work with them. In Beau's health analysis we see a lot of what was going on in mine and Bob's relationship. *'There is a great deal of secrecy that this one practices.'* He had that in his environment but also he was practicing it himself." At eight, Beau was practicing what he was learning.

"At this point Bob and I were still living life with our eyes closed. *'In the process of hiding these from others, this one developed a kind of insecurity.'* In many ways I was hiding a lot of who I was and what I thought with Bob. Honesty was not really part of our vocabulary. In fact, I was actually practicing dishonesty until I realized the value of complete communication. We've changed a lot. The intuitive reports have changed my life, my marriage, my parenting in ways I would never have suspected was possible.

"The Intuitive Health Analyses on children are invaluable. They are invaluable because a lot of times the child cannot tell you what's going on. They don't have the words. They don't have the experience. And it's a great tool for a parent to be able to understand and get greater understanding, not only for the child but for themselves."

"And then the lover"

"We see a fear of commitment within this one...."

Thus began Christine's husband's analysis. Just as an Intuitive Health Analysis on a child reflects the family, analyses conducted for two individuals who are married to each other can tell as much about their union as about themselves.

"When I heard my husband's health analysis I laughed to myself. I knew very well how he resisted committing to times and dates. It was often a source of frustration for me. I wondered if he would agree to the information that was presented. I knew he was going through a time of evaluation in his life and I hoped this would give him some clarity."

The opening of Andrew's reading described his mental state in this way:

> *We see a fear of commitment within this one. We see that this one battles within the Self concerning what this one wants, what this one believes and what this one will hold holy. We do see that this one harbors a fear that if this one commits the Self to a particular belief or a particular goal or a particular action that this one will then become trapped and lose freedom. Would suggest to this one that it is in this one deciding what this one wants, what this one believes, what this one stands for and then committing the Self to this through action that this one will discover this one's Self, this one will discover this one's creative ability and this one will then be free to create what this one desires based upon this kind of Self discovery. Would suggest to this one to practice this.*

The analysis was to the point, highlighting what Christine could readily see and aiding her to understand what before was an enigma to her. She wanted Andrew to benefit from what he heard at least as much as she was. "I believed in these reports but this was his first one." She was unsure that he would see as much truth in the analysis as she did. The verification began with what was obvious to her as a professional massage therapist:

> *We see that there is a great amount of muscular tension that occurs in the area of the head, neck and shoulders. We see that this relates to the fear of commitment and the accompanying burden that this one often ascribes to it. Would suggest massage, would suggest exercises in which this one rotates the neck and shrugs the shoulders and rotates the shoulders forward and back.*

Without a doubt they both knew Andrew carried tension in his upper body. Learning why was freeing.

To Christine's delight and surprise, "over the following months he did indeed decide to make some dramatic changes in jobs and location." Following a lifelong dream, Christine had moved an hour away from their home for a year of schooling, and Andrew decided to fulfill one of his dreams during that year. He moved from the Midwest to the northwestern states where the opportunity was present.

Christine was uneasy, but she knew she needed to be as giving as her husband was with her. "For me, hearing his analysis aided me to have objectivity and compassion." Andrew's analysis described how his thoughts were affecting his emotional state:

> *We see that within the emotional system that this one does have a capacity for enthusiasm and this can be used very productively when this one does have a goal. We see, however, that this one becomes very aloof emotionally when this one is called upon to draw forth this one's deeper Self. We see that once again this is related to the fear that this one will lose freedom if this one attaches the Self emotionally to a particular person, place or thing. Would suggest to this one that the freedom that this one desires will come from this one choosing how this one wants to use the emotions and express the Self emotionally. (1-31-95-LJC-4)*

Enthusiasm was part of what had initially attracted Christine to Andrew. He could make her laugh. In the years they had known one another, they had grown comfortable together. The intuitive analysis enabled her to let her husband go to pursue his dream, with the hope that he would accomplish what he wanted, even while she wrestled with her own imagined fears of abandonment.

"Four months after my husband's analysis was done I had a health analysis also. When I heard mine the first time I laughed out loud." The opening line said it all.

We see within this one there is a need for commitment.

"The mental attitudes were so similar! For Andrew a fear of commitment. For me, a need for commitment." The reason they had been attracted to one another revolved around the same characteristic, the ability to see something through to a point of conclusion. Just as the sameness drew them together, it also pulled them apart. "One of my friends asked jokingly why we ever got married. I answered, 'We wanted to learn about commitment.' That soul desire was obvious to me now." Because Christine wanted commitment she was much more prepared to embrace it than her husband. It was because Christine thought it was time for her and Andrew to do something – either get married or change somehow – that they had formalized their live-in association. In her analysis this was described as vacillation:

> ...*We see that for a long period of time this one has built awareness of this one's desires, this one's belief, this one's values and what this one believes to be most important in life. We see, however, that in regard to this one's activity this one vacillates and that when this one is insecure about this one's ability to truly accomplish what this wants and what this one values that this one pretends to the Self that this one does not really want this. Would suggest to this one that it is time for this one to face this pretense and to eliminate this line of thinking. For we see that this one wastes much time and much energy. This one's creativity and intelligence is therefore diminished. Would suggest to this one that this one commit the Self to what this one wants and direct the mind toward how this one can fulfill this in ever-growing ways rather than even questioning whether this is truth or not.*

Christine had a tendency to talk herself into or out of things. Experiences in her life had revealed to her a higher purpose, she did not yet know how to live this purpose. Discovering that living an ideal *is* commitment is what would bring her the fulfillment she craved. But the journey toward this realization was at times difficult:

> *We see within the emotional system that this one oftentimes views the emotions as being restrictive. We see that there are times when this one attempts to bypass the emotions. We see that there are other times when this one becomes completely consumed by them. Would suggest to this one that this one learn how to use emotion to cause this one's ideas to be brought forth in a very brilliant manner. We do see that this one has the capacity to be visionary and we see that using the emotions to bring this forward would aid this one in removing the doubt that this one holds on to. We see that much of the time when this one becomes consumed by the emotions is when this one is attempting to hold back and to repress the power of what this one truly desires. (5-30-95-LJC-4)*

Christine's conflicts were manifesting in her body primarily in the endocrine system; the adrenals, thyroid, and reproductive organs. The mental vacillation and emotional repression were the root of menstrual irregularities. When she asked what she could do to clear her face of acne, physical symptomatic suggestions were given only after the reader addressed the cause: *"this one needs to commit the Self to who this one wants to be."*

In Christine's and Andrew's case Intuitive Health Analyses became more than health reports, they were used to deal with important issues that affected their marriage. Christine says, "I often study these readings side by side. It still amazes me how parallel the mental, emotional and physical systems are. I appreciate the time and energy I have put forth to identify my values and beliefs. In many ways I see my husband still struggles with that.

"We have made changes in how we relate as a result of these reports. More so, however, we understand each other. It is like the adage when you point your finger at someone else there are three pointing back at you. Often our conflicts and misunderstandings centered on whether we were being true to our word – committed. The insights our analyses provided gave us a means of identifying our own attitudes. From this we began to explore the changes we wanted to make. What started as individual endeavors with individual health analyses has ended up to be one of the best things to happen in our marriage."

Lover or Soldier? Perhaps Both

Sharka Glet's reality lies somewhere between Shakespeare's definition of lover and soldier. She at once exemplifies a love of life, a love of her art, a love of self, and the struggle for recognition, accomplishment, and redemption.

Sharka was born in Czechoslovakia, now Czech Republic, a half century ago. She has firsthand experience of communist and republican forms of government, for she has lived in the United States for over two decades. She is an artist trained at the finest art institute in her native Prague, a wife, mother, business partner, teacher. Over the past decade she has requested yearly Intuitive Health Analyses, not so much for her physical state and well-being but to help her make sense of the many reactions her experience has provoked in her consciousness. For Sharka the health analyses bring a fresh, objective viewpoint that fosters Self examination and nurtures wisdom.

With her characteristic creative flair, Sharka researched her readings "to see the connection between my attitudes and fulfilling my life purpose." What she discovered reveals as much about the breadth of the Intuitive Health Analysis as it does about her personally.

"I know my Soul chose my Aries sun sign to learn something special. The challenge of the Aries influence is to build the identity of the Self as a creator. People with Aries sun signs usually have a very strong dominating ego. I understand the ego to be the reflection of the individual degree of awareness of understandings about creation. These understandings are held in our souls, stored in what is termed the Subconscious Mind.

"The function of the ego is to motivate the individual to create in the physical world by fulfilling his desires so more can be learned about creation and added to the soul's storehouse. The Conscious Ego uses the five senses to point out desires. We want what looks, smells, tastes, sounds or feels good. Because the ego is the reflection of the degree of individual awareness, our ego also knows awareness about the areas of creation which are lacking. According to that awareness the ego points to us the things in the physical world we want. In other words every desire we have gives us an opportunity to learn some missing piece about creation to expand our awareness.

"Everybody has different desires because we all have different degrees and different qualities of understandings about creation. For example: I always wanted to be famous and I used to think that everybody wants to be famous. To my surprise I found out that it was not true. To me it would feel good to be famous because of a lot of attention and probably money. Wanting to be famous was that sensually stimulated desire by my ego. The opportunity to learn when this desire is fulfilled is about honest communication.

"In order to be famous you need to be unique in the area of your expertise which you want to give. Everybody is a unique individual already because of the different sum of understandings in every individual soul. To be unique means you need to learn to be aware of those understandings, strengths, skills, talents and qualities, and to be able to communicate them honestly to the world. The skill to be able to give of yourself honestly is inevitable. [A] Famous person usually meets a lot of people so there is also a great opportunity to communicate verbally. Communication is a very important skill in learning about creation.

"We create with our thoughts. It is important to be able to formulate clear thought images in order to be able to create what we want. Through describing those mental images to others we can learn to be more clear and honest in our thinking and expressions each time we do that. I was a very shy person. I certainly needed to learn verbal communication. I am an artist and I chose to communicate only through my art for many years. I was hiding from verbal communication because I thought that I have nothing to say that anybody would be interested to hear. Because of my worthless attitude I greatly postponed practicing and learning verbal communication. Learning honest communication is my life purpose, it is the learning I need to add to my understanding about creation. That's why my ego wanted me to become famous.

"Before I had my first Intuitive Health Analysis I started to learn metaphysics in the School of Metaphysics. A large part of the learning is to share experiences in the class. I chose to print from my ten reports the parts which show my attitudes dealing with my ego during my interacting

with people and learning the honest communication.
    "Ego related attitudes in my first reading:

We see that in many ways this one holds on to a type of sadness and a type of depression. We see that this is due to this one's awareness. This one seems unable to please or to change this one's environment. (3-2-87-GBM-1)

"The reading describes my attitude trying to change the environment by taking responsibility for others. I even thought that I need to educate myself more to do that. I was doing things for people in order to help them and then I was unhappy when they were not grateful for it. My giving was conditional and so very egotistical. I started to use my Ego motivations to recognize my desires. I focused on fulfilling my desires and changing myself instead of trying to change others.
    "Ego related attitudes in my second reading:

There are many ideas that this one has as to how to be in control of this one's life. We see the difficulty however is that this one switches back and forth from this one trying to control others to trying to remove the self completely from the picture, condition, or circumstance. These two extremes leave this one irritated or impassioned with herself and others. (10-28-87-GBM-1)

"At this point of my life I made progress in communicating with people and I built some confidence through practicing it. I realized my great need to keep improving in self expression through verbal communication. I have recognized that verbal communication is more important for me to learn than expressing as an artist by painting. Simply because I didn't know how to do it yet.
    "I improved in having courage to speak but my interactions with others were most of the time forceful. I was telling people what to do and reacting when they told me what to do. I used to think that the solution is to do what I want to do and let them do what they want to do. That was the way I either tried to manipulate others or remove myself from the picture. I was listening to my ego which was trying to tell me that control is in controlling the outside instead of the inside environment. I started to learn consistency in making decisions to fulfill my desires and act upon them

consistently in order to be in control from inside.

"Ego related attitudes in my third reading:

This one is very upset when this one thinks that other people are disrespecting the self. It is not this one's problem when other people disrespect this one. It is a respect problem of her own. (9-12-89-CM-1)

"I took more steps in improving my self expression. I also kept educating myself in metaphysics and disciplining my mind. I became an instructor teaching metaphysics. This position gave me a great opportunity to practice verbal communication and to learn to give of myself.

"This analysis points out how I was disrespecting myself and others by being irresponsible in my thinking. I was avoiding completing my thinking process and actions by jumping to another thought before finishing the first one. I did it because my attention was upon physical things only, trying to do more physical tasks at the same time. My attention was on the physical accomplishments pointed by ego instead of being on what I was learning through accomplishment. I began to realize that the learning I craved occurs only from creation which is completed.

"Ego related attitudes in my fourth reading:

We see that this one's confusion in this period of time is based upon the attention this one wants to get from others, and changing this one's communication in order to gain approval from others. (5-1-90-CM-1)

"In order to be a better teacher I needed to be more honest. I was afraid that people wouldn't like me if I told them what I thought. My attention was on me instead of on aiding my students. I focused on learning to tell the truth as I see it.

"Ego related attitudes in my fifth report:

We see for this one to have a tendency to imagine limitations revolving around sensory experiences, and we see that this does result in this one refusing to see, refusing to hear, and refusing to experience with the senses. (9-26-90-CM-1)

"From this analysis I learned that in order to perceive someone else's need, I need to focus my mind and listen with all my senses. Then I am able to receive the truth and respond in communicating it to them. This is the means by which I am able to aid others.

"Ego related attitudes in my sixth report:

We see some insecurity that this one does contemplate often particularly when situations arise that are unexpected or that are new. This one's insecurity at the present time period is more in terms of how others view this one rather than how this one views the Self. (5-8-91-BGO-5)

"At this point in my life I kept improving in my speaking endeavors. I even gave several lectures to large groups of people. Some of these lectures were successful. Because I still continued a lot of times holding my attitude on worrying what people think of me, many times I misused my imagination, imaging the embarrassed situations. That's how I caused them to manifest. When what I imaged happened, I became even more afraid that it would happen again. I got myself in a vicious circle. This analysis helped me to realize what I was doing and start to imagine myself communicating successfully each time, imagining my desires instead of fears.

"Ego related attitudes in my seventh report:

This one has taken on the problems of other people, and we see that this one feels a sense of responsibility in solving their situations for them. We see that in the process this one has lost sight of the identity of the self and has become very critical of others. (3-13-92-BGC-6)

"I always cared for my students but I needed to admit that I was attached to them trying to solve their problems. After reading this analysis I realized the necessity to learn to focus on teaching them to reason and to solve their own problems.

"Ego related attitudes in my eighth reading:

We see difficulty in this one being unable to embrace new experiences or new learning. We see that much of this arises from insecurity. This one has a tendency to hold onto people, places, and things of the past that really serve no valuable purpose for this one in the present existence. (2-9-93-BGC-7)

"This reading made me realize that I still many times continued looking for security in the physical accomplishments instead of in my mental skills and strength. That's why I was becoming attached to the past, being afraid to change what was comfortable. Intellectually I knew all physical things are temporary that's why this attachment caused even more insecurity. I have realized that I have a very good imagination that I can create situations I want in my life. My artistic capabilities were demonstrated as if my life were the canvas. I started to see the security in my imagination instead of people or things outside of me, in some cases not even in my life any longer.

"Ego related attitudes in my ninth reading:

We see that this one does employ creative thinking in many different areas of this one's life and though this one has expanded this one's realm of thinking, this one only feels secure in doing this alone and when involved in artistic endeavors. When in action with others this one looses the sense of centeredness. This one's attention is simply moved to how she appears to others, how she is being received by others. We see that this one expects rejection from them since she is rejecting herself. (9-21-93-BGC-1)

"I realized how learning mental skills in communicating verbally helped me greatly in understanding my artistic expression. I have improved tremendously as an artist. This analysis helped me to realize that I know how to be centered when I paint. I started being more attentive to my state of mind while painting and endeavored to apply this understanding when interacting with others. Almost immediately I felt a difference. It took longer to really cultivate it.

"Ego related attitudes in my tenth report:

We see that although this one thinks that this one is thinking of others, this one's entire thinking revolves around the self and in what way this one can obtain what this one desires. (12-6-94-LJC-2)

"With this analysis I finally realized that my insecurity, whether caused by a fear of being embarrassed or worrying about others' ideas of me, is very selfish. The pieces began to fall into place. My desire always was to help people. I needed to admit that I was not capable of doing it without controlling my ego.

"I had to realize that even that I had come a long way in my speaking improvements I still needed to learn to communicate honestly. My attitude most of the time was selfish and went like: 'People are here for my learning.' I started to create a new thought 'I am here for people.'

"This new thinking gave me a peace, excitement, and sense of worthiness. Telling people what they need to hear regardless of what they would think of me brought me freedom and respect from others because I was becoming honest with myself.

"I don't think I would be able to hear, admit, and change my attitude without the benefit of these analyses. The physical information was valuable, but the intuitive insight concerning me, how I see myself and why, continues to be invaluable. I am very grateful also for my metaphysical study and to my teachers who are guiding me to be selfless in how I aid others and to fulfill my life purpose by doing it."

"Then a soldier"

One spring afternoon, Paul Blosser was returning home on a two-lane stretch of highway. A long day, he had run errands all over town and Paul knew he'd been pushing himself in general. For a moment Paul took his mind off the road and within seconds the back of the tractor-trailer truck he had been following was crunching and climbing the hood of his 1993 Ford pick-up. "The last thing I remember was reaching down to get my coffee mug, then the sound of glass breaking."

Paul walked away from the accident. One of the first things he did was schedule an Intuitive Health Analysis at the earliest available time.

Paul is well acquainted with Intuitive Health Analyses. He knew an analysis would tell him what he needed to know about the condition of his physical body, what kind of damage had been done and where. But more important to Paul was the insight it could bring concerning "why". This was not the first time he had been in a car accident. In fact it was his third in less than ten years. Paul understood these kinds of near-death experiences as etheric citations for change, omens. The first question he asked concerned the cause of his accident and the intuitive reporter replied, *"This has already been given."* So with Paul we start with his 1997 analysis just days following his accident:

> *We see a testing of this one's spirit being experienced at this time. We see that this one is evaluating the intentions of the Self in a different perspective than has been for quite some time. We see that there has been a catharsis in this one's attitudes of late and we see that there have been changes in regards to this one's level of commitment, this one's ability to image the Self and this one's desire... (4-10-97-BGC-1)*

Paul's life had become very full in the few years prior to this report, and since his last car accident. He owned his own computer consulting firm, traveled weekly, was married to a wonderful woman, was reconciling with his now-grown daughter, and devoted half his time to humanitarian service. It was only recently that he was beginning to appreciate what he had in his life. The reality of goodness in his life was a bit overwhelming. Gratitude was causing Paul to remember why he had wanted his life this way and to question if the same motives were still present or applicable, or even wanted.   This caused the *"catharsis."*

Previously it had been Paul's pattern to defeat himself, often rejecting the gifts life brought before even knowing what they were. With many physical desires fulfilled, Paul was at a place where he needed to change ingrained patterns of thinking, habits that made him question the longevity of his good fortune thereby ensuring its end. He was struggling with this, wanting to remain steadfast in the productive thinking that brought him the life he wanted yet being tempted to allow the old patterns to have dominion.

Paul had come farther in the last few years of his life than in all the years before. He knew he was ready for another step in awareness but he was dragging his feet. He hadn't given in to the negative, self-defeating tendencies, but they were knocking at his door. And so, before Paul could destroy with his fears what he had built, the opportunity to put everything in perspective arose:

> *We see that this has been shaken however in reaction to circum-stances outside the Self and we see that this one is having difficulty in holding onto the ideals that he had begun to form. We see that this is a pattern for this one and we see that this one has often allowed the will to remain weak and to lack the inner support necessary to elevate the awareness and to cause transformation in the Self. We see that this one needs to recognize that the power within the Self resides in the capacity for reason and we see that as this one would move away from pretense and intellectual ideas into wisdom and understanding that there would be the security that this one desires, there would be the strength that this one admires and the fortitude that this one covets.*
>
> *Would suggest that this one recognize the situations in the life as tests for these are indeed what they are. They are also signals inasmuch as they cause this one to evaluate, they cause this one to think more deeply and to become more committed. They do not exist to discredit this one, to discourage this one or to defeat this one,*

which has been this one's pattern of emotional reaction to adversity... (4-10-97-BGC-1)

It is probably odd to most people to see a car accident as an opportunity, but most who have lived to tell about the experience are changed by it. Facing death does bring life into perspective, no matter what the circumstances. This was true for Paul.

"I requested a health analysis from the School of Metaphysics for two reasons; 1) I wanted to know the mental cause of the accident and 2) I knew the analysis would provide the information I would need to achieve optimum health, mentally, emotionally and physically," Paul told me. "I was aware of unproductive thoughts I had in the past; self-defeating thoughts of anger, fear and disappointment. I specifically wanted greater insight to these, not realizing that it was my self-defeating perspective that was at the core of my accident.

"The reading revealed a *'testing of this one's spirit'* to cause me to evaluate, explore within myself and to think more deeply than I had in quite some time. I had two choices; I could choose to be a 'victim' and for my experience to be self-defeating, or I could choose to be a creator and for my experience to be a stimulus for me to be true to my ideas, ideals, and images.

"There had really been few opportunities in my life where I came face to face with adversity; I rarely studied in high school, but graduated with A's and B's. After high school, I did very well in the military, rising above my peers. I was the first member of my family to go to college and made good grades easily. None of these experiences gave me the opportunity to stretch or to push myself beyond anything more than physical limits.

"At the time of this accident, I was at a place in my life where I needed to go beyond my spiritual limits to achieve the *'security that this one desires, the strength that this one admires and the fortitude that this one covets.'* My analysis revealed that such situations *'do not exist to discredit this one, to discourage this one or to defeat this one.'*

"One of the keys in the reading is that *'life is a series of choices and that each is to be relished.'* Upon reviewing past intuitive analyses, this simple truth is one that had been eluding Paul for most of his life. A 1993 analysis described Paul's predominant mental attitude as anxious. His anxiety was *'produced from the separation that this one does promote in terms of this one's own self. We see that it manifests in regards to this one's relations with others.'* Those were hard days for Paul. He was working for someone else, alienated from his only child, and finding it difficult to cultivate long-standing relationships with others. It was the time period of a previous wreck where he fell asleep at the wheel, just yards from the rest stop ramp he was going to take, and plowed his car into the back of a flatbed truck. He walked away from that one too.

What robbed him in 1993 of realizing the truth about choice was a fear that made him see others as being against him: "*a fear that this one will not be able to change, that this one will not be able to cause intimate associations with others.*" That entire analysis described Paul's tendency to cause a separateness in his life, particularly in relationships with others. Aware of this, efforts to change it produced anxiety not rapport. The reading described it as *"fitful attempts at being able to produce intimacy and closeness with others without giving the self the benefit of closeness."*

Another analysis later in 1993 helped Paul to make strides in being comfortable and at peace with himself. It identified the cause of Paul's fears of intimacy as *"difficulty in establishing a kind of relationship or rapport with the inner self....this one is aware of many different means in which this one can create this rapport. We see that these need to be implemented with joy and with respect rather than with forceful actions to cause an immediate transformation." (4-1-93-BGC)* Paul took this advice to heart and turned his life around. His company and reconciling with his daughter began in 1993. He married a year later.

Four years later he may not have all the answers yet but his emotional progress is undeniable. That's why he could now be emotionally calm in expression even though inside he was reeling from all the implications of the wreck.

> *We see that this one's emotional state is outwardly calm but inwardly in turmoil and we see that it is this pretense, this dishonesty within the Self that is practiced over and over and it causes this one to not be able to trust the Self. It also causes this one the kind of disheartening that does defeat him time and time again. Would suggest that this one be willing to become much more direct and much more truthful with the Self mentally and emotionally so that*

this one can find the point of stability and commitment that he does desire... (4-10-97-BGC-1)

The same root problem was described in the 1993 analysis. Comparing the two emotional assessments reveals how far Paul had come in understanding his emotions: *"Emotionally, this one creates great strain. This is a pattern. It is perpetuated. It is intentionally repeated. It is a way that this one can feel alive without needing to confront the isolation. Would suggest this one learn how to distinguish between what is real and what is fantasy, what is permanent and what is temporary, what is needed and what is desired."* Paul at last could see what was defeating him time and again, the pretense. When you think you're looking death in the eye, all of a sudden whatever pretenses you had are gone. Physical pain does the same thing. It momentarily cleanses the mind of what is not real because it gives the mind no escape from the site of the pain. The following, an excerpt from a 1994 analysis, sheds light upon Paul's repeated brushes with death:

> *We see reticence in the mental system. We see that although this has changed in some forms, we see that it is still the primary reaction mentally that this one has to experiencing. We see that this is a deliberate pulling back and away from experience. We see that it is a reaction to anticipated pain and we see that this one goes to extreme lengths to protect the self from pain. We see it is not that this one does not experience discomfort or unpleasantness or pain, but it is that this one tries to hide this fact from others. We see that this then promotes a facade and a kind of attitude of hiding or refusing to reveal the self as this one would see it.*
>
> *Would suggest to this one that this one equally to pain does experience pleasure. Therefore would suggest that this one begin to reveal the pleasure that this one finds in life. We see this one does have the capability of having a most optimistic and encouraging attitude toward the self and others. It is this that this one needs to honestly build, rather than to feel that doing so would be in some way untruthful. We see that it is through the consistent effort of identifying and acting upon truth that this one will begin to transcend the pain and pleasure of temporal experience. (1-18-94-BGC)*

Only by transcending the body do we release attachment to the pain. Only by transcending his isolation did Paul begin to release his fear of people and himself. Now truth needed to become the center of Paul's thinking. And again the reminder that life is a choice. Paul could relinquish the facade he used as a fortress, freeing his true nature of optimism and encouragement to blossom. By utilizing the power of his mind, his capacity for creative thinking, he would give new guidance to his emotions, thus ending years of emotional pain.

> *We see that this one does become entrapped very easily in emotional reactions and then it does have its repercussions in the mental system. We see that this one is afraid of his own power emotionally and we see that this is part of the attempt upon the mental system to pull back, to hide. We see that this does not create understanding. It merely perpetuates this one's pain.*
>
> *Would suggest therefore for this one to become more aware of what is desired and to become more open to the manifestation of those desires. As this one would do so, this one would become more cognizant of the energies as they move through the emotions and would have less fear of them and more of a curiosity would develop in terms of the emotion's function. This attitude of curiosity would aid this one greatly mentally and emotionally.   (1-18-94-BGC-1)*

Paul heeded much of this analysis. Seriously studying the implications of what was being said, and seeking ways to enact the suggestions. In four years' time, the difference in Paul's awareness was apparent not only in the changes in his life but more importantly the changes in how he thinks of himself and others. This was clearly demonstrated in the following questions he posed during his 1997 analysis:

Q: "How can I deal with the fear, anger and disappointment within myself?"

> *Would suggest that this one discipline the mind to elevate the awareness to purposely view this physical occurrence in an entirely different light from what is this one's pattern. We see that all though it does have its repercussions and this one will indeed be responsible for them, that it is not a matter of the experience holding within it a form of intention. This is to say that the experience did not and*

does not determine how this one will think or react to it. This one is choosing to react in a fearful manner. This one is choosing to defeat the Self. It is not the situation that will defeat this one. Would suggest that this is the test that has been alluded to previously and suggestions have been given for alternative ways that this one can view what has occurred and can use it as a springboard towards elevating his own consciousness rather than dragging himself down...

Q: What is the greatest fear that this one has, the main fear?

Not being what this one portends to be. (4-10-97-BGC-1)

Paul had ceased projecting his fear onto others – the idea that others could hurt him if they discovered who he really was. This was Paul's old way of thinking whereby he surrendered control and centered his problem around others. Paul had made significant inroads into understanding himself, his motivations, and his strengths. This brought him home to the realization that he is the center of his universe. Now he could own his fear admitting that he was very close to resolving an inner battle of whether to give of himself or hide who he is.

Paul fought this battle for four decades, and it left its psychic impression upon his consciousness. Impressions that appeared repeatedly in intuitive readings. A key to winning the battle of despair appeared in the 1994 analysis. When Paul asked about his attitudes concerning money, wealth, and abundance this was the response:

This one has a tendency to dwell upon what this one does not want to occur and we see that these are areas which this one allows the dwelling to happen. It is part of this one's tendencies toward negative thinking, rather than building upon this one's ability to think in a positive, creative way.

Q: Any further suggestions for this entity in replacing the fear with courage and desire?

It is most important for this one to have faith in the self, to form a very strong belief in who this one is. (1-18-94-BGC-4)

Paul acted on many of the suggestions here. Creating physical success was an important step in his growth, and by 1997 what had been the goal was now a stepping stone toward something greater. In some ways Paul's belief in himself was fresh; tender and vulnerable. Like an Old Testament patriarch, there came a time when the power of that faith was tested.

This wreck was a manifestation of whatever fears and doubts Paul continued to maintain. Those thoughts of "who am I kidding?" "can I keep this up?" "I might as well give up now," remnants of his old self. They were ideas from another person who had increasingly less and less to do with the person Paul was becoming. The test was who would prevail during the tougher times, the old Paul or the new Paul.

Within a day or so after the wreck, Paul's bruises started to show and he was unable to move without considerable discomfort. He had gone from the wreck site to his chiropractor who had begun the physical repair work. His analysis described pre-existing conditions as well as those particularly linked to the physical trauma his body had endured. Although it does not give a universal description of what being in a car wreck will do to your body, this analysis does attest to the value of intuitive knowledge both for the mental/emotional insight and the description of the condition of the body following such a crises.

> *We see within the physical system that there has been upheaval that has occurred, particularly in regards to the endocrine system. There have been great amounts of hormones which have been released into this body within the recent past and it is causing repercussions throughout all the systems. There has been some bruising within internal organs; the right lung, the spleen and adrenal glands in particular. We see that these areas are under duress at the present time period and need healing.*
>
> *We see that there have been some secondary repercussions in the musculature of the body, but we see that much of the friction here is related to the hormones. It is important at this point for this one to be able to channel energy throughout the body, to keep the energy moving. We see that this one does have the capacity to direct the imagination in this regard. We see that this one is also aware of ways of physically moving the body to stimulate this kind of energy*

movement.

We see that the immune system is working diligently at the present time period for there are so many weakened areas of the body that there is susceptibility to bacterial and viral conditions. We see that although there are many types of substances that could be taken into the system, that the best release in the body would be found by ingesting large quantities of water. This would serve as a means to flush the system without adding any kind of substance which would need to be responded to by the body. Would suggest that, that referred to as lemon grass in the form of a tea or as an essential oil could provide a stimulus that would be very soothing to the body itself. Lavender would likewise produce this effect.

We see that there is a hairline fracture in several of the ribs on the right side of the body. We see that these can easily be repaired. We see that there has been some disruption of the way they are attached, however this too, with slight manipulation and with time will heal. We see that there has been some difficulty in the head plates, between the occipital portion and the parietal portion of the skull. Massage of the head, gentle massage would be stimulating, not only to the movement of this area but also the release of energy. Breathing, relaxed deep inhalations and exhalations, would also be helpful in the head area, as well as to the body as a whole.

We see that there has been stress in the muscles of the upper cervical and upper thoracic regions. Massage of these tissues would be helpful in aiding there to be a rebuilding of the strength which would hold the vertebrae in place and support the head without adverse tension. We see that there is a tendency for subluxation in the 4th, 5th and 6th thoracic (vertebra). There is also a tendency for difficulty in the upper lumbar area and a kind of static that occurs in the sacral region. We see that acupuncture could be helpful in these areas for they are of considerable duration. We see that they do contribute to some difficulty in energy flowing directly in to the legs and the digestive system, particularly the stomach.

We see that there has been ulcerations in the stomach and we see that this is due to a bacterial condition. We see that the use of allicin which is found in fresh garlic would be very helpful in eliminating the bacteria from the system. We see that there have been substances taken into the body at times which have disrupted the digestive tract in an attempt to balance it when in effect it has created more imbalance and we see there is a need for this to be

changed as it causes greater pressure and burden on the body
without addressing what is the difficulty. We see that even before
the bruising of the adrenals, there was some deterioration of
function here. There is also some sluggishness in the thyroid and
some sporadic movement in the pituitary. We see that this is due to
the way in which this one thinks and utilizes the will in the ways that
have already been described. This is all.   (4-10-97-BGC-1)

Each of Paul's analyses cited imbalances in the endocrine function, stomach problems, and varying spinal difficulties. These were the areas that continued to be stressed by the attitudes described. Their appearance once again in this analysis pointed to the continued call to meet creative potential.

Paul was present during this analysis and he asked a number of questions ranging from physical ones about the lymph glands to ones concerning his greatest anger. Without hesitation or apology, Paul addressed a most critical issue: "sometimes I have thoughts of giving up, thinking that a particular goal isn't worth it. I think this leads to disappointment in myself. How can I change this way of thinking?"

This is very true and we see that when this occurs, there are
situations that arise in this one's life that test this one's observa-
tions. Likewise, when this one becomes motivated to move forward,
something that this one considers a test will arise in one form or
another and we see that this is a repeated pattern. It is the means
by which this one offers the Self an opportunity to evaluate his own
identity, to evaluate who he is, why he exists and where he is going.
We see that this has not been the way that this one has responded
for the most part to these kinds of challenges in his life, but it is what
this one can develop and it is what would give this one the spiritual
upliftment and the fulfillment that he very much craves. We see that
it is a matter of this one's willingness. We see that this one needs to
deeply internalize into his consciousness that 'Life is a series of
choices' and that until this one recognizes this fully and recognizes
that the choices are his own to be made and to be relished this one
will continue to view the situations as a means to defeat his own
awareness of his inner urges. (4-10-97-BGC-1)

The final suggestions of Paul's analysis were for his soul growth and spiritual development. The response holds universal meaning for any soldier of life. It is perhaps the reason we fight so hard to live a complete and satisfying life: *"Would suggest that this one endeavor at this time to support himself in his best efforts – forsaking all other patterns which might defeat this."*

"And then the justice"

The capacity for self-revelation exists in each of us.
It is a tendency for man to try to come to this point of awareness through intellect only, by watching, judging, and concluding with very little experiencing. This superficial approach to life produces restlessness and dissatisfaction because it ignores personal desires and fails to fulfill inner soul urges for growth. Undisciplined, intellectualism is also the breeding ground for insecurity. Disciplined, the intellect begins the journey toward fulfillment by sparking the imagination which fuels the will to succeed. This eventually culminates in the direct grasp of Truth.

Such a life lesson is addressed in this analysis done for Teresa Martin, a medical lab technician from Chicago:

> We see confusion in the mental system that arises in this one's insecurity and not knowing the choices that can be made for action that will implement this one's ideas. We see that this one believes the difficulty is in the decision making, when in reality this one's difficulty is in the imaging fully and completely what is desired to be. We see that there is a need for this one to purposefully exercise the complete use of the imagination to incorporate all senses in the use of the mental attention and to direct it with one-pointed focus.
>
> This one becomes distracted very easily and therefore creates very vague ideas, which then this one can incompletely act upon. We see that this one becomes distracted in thoughts that it is what this one is or is not doing physically in terms of action that causes this one's success or failure. When in reality it is what this one is or is not doing in terms of the imagination that produces this. Would suggest that adjustments be made.
>
> We see that as a result this one finds that the emotions are incomplete in their expression and in this one's ability to understand them. We see that this one therefore tends to run away from

the emotions, to ignore them, or hide them or avoid them at all costs. We see that this creates great pain in this one. We see that this one attempts to hide the pain by becoming somewhat impervious and we see that this merely prolongs this one's distress rather than to aid in its resolve.

Would therefore suggest to this one to begin to recognize that the full expression of what this one perceives will aid this one and will accelerate the ability to identify the emotions and to understand them for what they are. This one tends to confuse objectivity and indifference. This one needs to learn how to distinguish the two and how to become truly objective while in action rather than attempt to remove the Self through indifference.

We see within the physical body that there is difficulty in the commands from the thinking reaching the body. Therefore the body tends to be sluggish in its functioning. It tends to hold on to fat that it does not require. It tends to hold onto fluid that is does not need, it tends to hold onto dead tissue which is no longer required by the organs of the physical body. We see that much of the state of the body in the present is a state of stagnancy in terms of its functioning.

We see that the internal organs for the most part do perform their function but it is always under duress because these areas are always being pulled down by the excess that is held in the physical frame. Therefore there is the need for this one to release; to release thinking, to release emotion, to release waste physically. This will only be accomplished as this one involves the Self through the use of the imagination with the present moment and with producing the future that this one desires. This action will enable this one to place the past in proper perspective rather than hold onto it for fear that it might be lost.

We see that there could be some benefit derived from the stimulation of the major acupuncture meridians along the spinal column particularly involving that referred to as the ida and pingala. We see that there would be some benefit derived from chiropractic or osteopathic attention as well for the spinal column does tend to be somewhat malformed or malshaped and there is a tendency for the frontal head plates to be misaligned. This is all....
(1-18-94-BGC-1)

"All of my life I had many ideas of how things could be better. I recall hearing my parents speak about their concerns about family matters;

financial situations, coordinating schedules, expanding our farm by purchasing additional property or equipment. Over the years, this has been a common theme; I could always see how things could be made better. I was pretty insecure most of my life regarding communication of my ideas, so over time, I communicated these less and less. In my mind though I knew the ideas would work. What developed was a kind of arrogance which was actually a form of dishonesty. The ideas that I placed so much value in were worthless if they never manifested.

"At the time I had this reading I was beginning to realize this. I had studied Applied Metaphysics for five years and had received a tremendous amount of information. I had so much information in my brain, information that was supposed to hold the keys to supernormal creative abilities. I knew that I had the information, but there was something missing in terms of how I used it. And I really wanted to figure out how to use it.

"Since I knew I already had a good grasp of formulating ideas, I thought the missing piece in my ability to create my desires was in the implementation of steps of creation. So I resolved to learn this. But in my attempt to do so, I compensated too much and focused primarily on the activity, and lost sight of the skills in imaging I had.

"The confusion as spoken of in the reading was a result of focusing too much on activity. Metaphysics is not something you apply only once in a while, it's intended to be a part of daily life. The mind is very powerful and facilitates everything we do. It's not something you start up one moment and then shut down when you do some action. The mind is thought in action.

"What occurred in my attitudes and in my mind was like swirling around lots of thoughts, much like the motion of a whirlwind, spinning round and round in the same space. My thoughts were constantly reviewing what worked, what didn't work, what others had said or done. My thoughts were in constant motion, but without direction. I sought solutions in activity rather than imagining what I really desired, or who I really wanted to become through the activities I involved myself in. Over time this lack of direction through clear imaging manifested in my body in which the energy was becoming very sluggish. There were many energy blockages, meaning the flow to organs and tissues was depleted. Physically this manifested as extreme tiredness, sluggishness in my digestive system, and a build up of toxins, with difficulty releasing waste products completely.

What I was doing with my thoughts was similar to driving a car with the foot on the accelerator and brake simultaneously. My mind was constantly moving but without direction.

"One of the suggestions given by the intuitive reporter was to have stimulation of the acupuncture meridians along the spinal column particularly the ida and pingala. When I visited my chiropractor, upon examination she explained that my parasympathetic and sympathetic nervous systems were both out of balance. She said this was somewhat unusual to have both out of balance, as they tend to operate alternatively.

"I saw my chiropractor quite regularly for some time. She balanced the energy flows along the spinal column and I balanced my thinking. I began writing a dissertation which I'd thought about for a long time. I wanted to use this as a way to bring my thoughts completely out into the physical one step at a time. I started by outlining the chapters based on what I believed people needed to know the most about my topic which was centered around viewing conditions and circumstances as opportunity rather than as a problem. Any situation we find troublesome may be a golden opportunity to discover something important about ourselves, depending on how you look at it. Even illness can be a blessing in disguise if it causes you to 'wake up' and appreciate life more and discover the unhealthy attitudes that led to the disease in the first place. Then you change them.

"I formed the basic idea for chapter one by asking myself the question; 'What was the most important thing for people to realize if they were to view the existing conditions, good or bad, as an opportunity rather than seeing themselves as being out of control?' Then I planned the next thing people would need to know and formulated this idea for the second chapter. Through this process I outlined the entire dissertation and then set about filling in the details. The guiding principle I used was that every word would be used purposefully to illustrate the primary thought the dissertation was built around. It was in this way that I came to understand how to physically manifest a creation rather than simply thinking about it over and over again. A dissertation, book or any written composition is a collection of words put together to express an idea or thought. All I needed to do was to focus in the present to determine what detail to add to.

"This process aided me to learn to give direction to my thoughts. Imagining clearly within my mind the next step and then implementing that step. This is how any creation occurs from the tallest building to the most luscious dessert. I discovered how to create in steps and this was an important foundation for a belief I now hold. I can do anything I put my mind to."

Each Intuitive Health Analysis details wholistic health, but even more so it presents the querent with a description of the lesson he or she is to learn. Sometimes that lesson involves issues spanning the lifetime, sometimes it revolves around something new in the person's life. Whichever the lesson is timely. Assimilating the ideas given deepens self-understanding in ways few other experiences can. Some have said that in ten minutes what they received in a health analysis surpassed years of therapy. They are remarkable because the people they describe are remarkable.

Intuitive Health Analyses describe what one person is doing with his or her mind and how that thinking affects the body. To perceive how one person's consciousness molds the human body is awesome. What it tell us about who we are and what we are capable of as a species is inspiring. Consider the following insights into a universal experience for every female whose life spans half a century.

"*I had heard a comment about menopause* from an analysis years ago which had sparked my curiosity about this change," says Elizabeth Stewart. "It had said that during menopause the way creative energy is used changes. The analysis didn't describe what kind of change would occur but that there is a change in the way creative energy is used.

"Physically, creative energy during the child-bearing years is being used for the reproduction and nurturing of another physical being. There are many activities going on in a woman's body during the monthly cycles: activity in the pituitary gland, hypothalamus, the adrenals and reproductive organs, the manufacturing of a balance of estrogen and progesterone and the communication between all these different glands, organs, and systems. Although this is a physical cycle in the body the use of creative energy is still needed to make it happen.

"When these cycles begin to shut down it doesn't mean a woman loses this creative energy. In fact, it means the creative energy once needed to perpetuate the child-bearing cycle is available for other uses. This report had sparked my curiosity about what I would experience as I approached menopause and the energies began to shift in my body.

"When I received my analysis I was astounded at what I heard.

We see within the physical system there is movement that is occurring within the endocrine system that is irregular. There is a change that is occurring in the levels of estrogen and progesterone in this body. There are changes that are occurring in the reproductive system, the pituitary, the hypothalamus, the adrenals. (3-1-97-LJC-1)

"The changes were not only occurring in the reproductive organs and hormone levels but the pituitary, adrenals and hypothalamus too! The pituitary is a master gland of the physical body. On a metaphysical level, the area where the pituitary can be found is the area where an energy transformer or chakra is also found. The brow chakra is associated with the pituitary gland and works directly with energies of insight and spiritual perception. The hypothalamus works alongside the pituitary, kind of like its right hand man, producing some of the hormones that the pituitary sends to the body. It is also the seat of the emotions and autonomic nervous system. The adrenal gland also works with the autonomic nervous system. The autonomic nervous system is what governs all the involuntary functions of the body like breathing, digestion, heart rate and so on. Metaphysically these organs are governed by the subconscious mind. So the pituitary, hypothalamus and adrenal glands all work in direct relationship to the subconscious mind, the seat of the soul and intuition."

"When I heard about these glands my thought was, 'What does God have in store for me to do for the rest of my life?' The relationship between the conscious and subconscious minds was changing. This was the change in the energies I had heard about in another woman's analysis years before!"

As a minister and healer, Elizabeth had become well-versed in wholistic health. Her extensive knowledge now had a place to be applied in her own life, a place to be utilized for her own deeper understanding.

"The energies once used to produce during the adult years were now being directed to cause there to be a reflection of the life, a drawing together of experiences into wisdom, of insight into what one has become through the journey of life. There is a maturity of thought that one can give the world and to the Self. I knew this change wasn't unique to my own physical body and being, but universal for all women and probably men too. But I had received this information and embraced it as a covenant with my higher Self. There was something very purposeful laid out for me to do for the rest of my life, and my mind and body were beginning to prepare for it."

Elizabeth had been courting this awareness throughout her forties. I remember several years previous to this Elizabeth would be preoccupied, slightly scattered, much to her consternation. Such distraction was unwelcomed in her life, and it worried her. She even began wondering if this was a first sign of what might later develop into senility, Alzheimer's disease. An analysis done in 1993 answered her questions about this, and much more:

> *We see austerity in the mental system that this one uses against the self as a kind of punishment. We see...this one finds the self lacking in comparison with what this one is able to imagine. We see that part of this is due to a lack of utilization of will, but much of it is in regards to this one's need to image the self in actions that this one finds admirable.*
>
> *We see that there are many times when this one does not take time to think. In many ways this one is trying to pretend that she is spiritual but in the everyday activities and actions this idea is not alive. We see that there has been much striving to change this but it has been made into a problem or a burden or a difficulty instead of a joy. We see that this one has been attempting to find a source of joy and we see that as this one releases the severity in this one's thinking, in this one's judgements, in this one's assessment of herself, in this one's delineation of right and wrong – as this is replaced with a sense of openness, a sense of expansiveness, a sense of discovery, then this one will begin to realize the beauty in everyday occurrences... (4-17-93-BGC-6)*

Elizabeth's search for completeness, for wholeness, for peace, was often a struggle that was disrupting the functioning of her brain:

> *...We see that there is a hypersensitivity that tends to occur in the limbic system and it does interfere with the teleplay between the pituitary and hypothalamus. We see that this then does in turn affect the functioning of the brain and there are times when this one finds*

*that the nervous system does not seem to working appropriately.
There is a need for vitamin B complex particularly B6 to be added
as a supplement to this one's diet. Would suggest the utilization of
dong quai and ginko biloba would be helpful as well in a greater
functioning of the brain and nervous system. (4-17-93-BGC-6)*

This analysis went even further. It described in detail both the mind pattern
that was causing Elizabeth's struggle and the kind of thinking that would
create a new pattern. The awarenesses that would, a few short years,
blossom in Elizabeth foreshadowed here:

*There is a need for this one to become more invested in this one's
life. We see that this one has moved the self to a position of
importance in many different areas to many different people. We
see that there are ways in which this one casts doubt upon this and
therefore degrades what her offerings are. It is time that this one
move past this denigration and begin to assume a kind of respectful
office in terms of how she thinks of herself and how she thinks of
other people. As this one is willing to do so, there would be then a
willingness to embrace each moment. This one needs to have this
kind of consciousness in order for her to cause the brain to work
completely. (4-17-93-BGC-6)*

With her 1997 analysis Elizabeth became acutely aware of a
synthesis occurring deep in her consciousness, unlike any she had known
before and of the nature she had craved all her life.

"I began to think that maybe I am one of those late bloomers who
really doesn't come into their own until late in life. There is a quiet beauty
about autumn. The earth is quieting down from the hot summer. Days and
nights are cooler. The insects, having laid their eggs are dying; the birds are
migrating and many animals are seeking a nest for hibernation. The
brilliant gold and red plumage on the trees is a reminder that, yes, there is
creation in the midst of this waning autumn season.

"The brilliance when the leaves begin to change color is the
brilliance I have to look forward to in my own life."

"The sixth age shifts"

Al Rohrer is approaching his eighth decade of life. He is to date the oldest person on record to receive a Doctorate in Metaphysics from the School of Metaphysics. He is a testimony to the many benefits of applying metaphysics in your life. His character is impeccable, his humor sly, and his humbleness admirable. As for physical stamina, he can run rings around youngsters a quarter his age.

In 1993, Al received an Intuitive Health Analysis that would change his life...

> *We see a kind of self effacing which occurs within the mental system. We see that this is a very pronounced, nourished and practiced way of viewing the self that affects all of this one's life.*

"I put the essence of my health reading in two words: self-effacing. These two words describe the story of much of my life, for I have held an image of unworthiness in my mind for many years." The analysis went on to describe what he knew about myself but had difficulty putting into words.

> *...We see that this one continually puts himself down. We see that this results in this one covering up the strength of the self and, in this one's thinking, does absolve the self of responsibility.*
>
> *We see this one has spent much of his existence in trying to be reliable, dependable, responsible according to what this one believed is expected of him, and in that way he has been very dependent upon others to supply him with discipline.*

It was true. Al had led a very full life. Born in 1919 in a German-speaking Swiss settlement in the Mississippi River hills, all four of Al's grandparents migrated from Switzerland. Acceptable behavior and the need to act in certain ways was instilled in him by his family. He knew what was expected of him and he spent his life striving to do his duty. He owned his own business for decades, married, raised six children, served God and man in his church and was a pillar in the community. He was indeed reliable, dependable and responsible according to what he thought others wanted from him. He gave more thought to what others might think than to what he thought and this was the crux of his difficulty in the senior years of his life.

> *We see that this has left this one however without a sense of internal discipline, without a sense of internal structure, and with a lack of understanding of the value of what this one has accomplished in this one's discipline and responsibility. We see that this one has spent much time lying to the self concerning this and we see that this has been done in that this one will credit and blame others for why this one is responsible or irresponsible rather than this one accepting the reality of his own choice. Would suggest to this one that by seeing his mind to recognize the caliber, the quality, the construction of his own way of thinking, and not falling into attaching this to someone outside of himself, this one will begin to reveal the fact of the value of the life that this one has lived. We see that it is only this one that is blinding the self to this. (4-17-93-BGC-M)*

The wealth of Al's life is truly astounding to others, even when he takes it for granted. One collection of memories that reveal the kind of person Al is, the caliber and quality of his thinking, revolve around Immanuel Magomolia.

Al writes, "In 1966, a black Carthage College student who had come here from Tanzania, Africa, spoke to the Kenosha, Wisconsin Lions Club. I wanted to know more about Immanuel's country and its people, so my wife and I invited him to our home for Sunday dinner. He had come to Carthage College under the auspices of the Lutheran Church to get a college education, and his goal was to become a medical missionary. Since he already had Lutheran training in Africa, we asked our pastor if Immanuel could deliver the sermon some Sunday, and the arrangements were made for the following month.

"Immanuel was born in Ntawike, Tanzania, where his father, Zakayo, (from the biblical Zacchaeus) had a small banana farm. Immanuel belonged to the Bantu Tribe, and spoke Swahili, a language of Arabic derivation. He was educated at a Lutheran School which was operated by missionaries from Minneapolis, Minnesota. It was called a 'Bush School' and was an eight mile walk from his home. The building was made of mud blocks and had a corrugated tin roof and a dirt floor.

"In the spring of 1969, our family decided to use our Easter vacation to tour the warmer south. We planned to go through Illinois, Missouri, Arkansas and Louisiana– destination, New Orleans. Immanuel expressed a desire to see the south, so we invited him along. We were happy to have another driver so that we could use two cars, since we were bringing our six children, ages three to 17. Immanuel then asked whether he could bring Darleen, a white college friend.

"Although we had been down south on our honeymoon in 1951, and had seen the 'whites only' signs on the water fountains and restrooms, we felt sure that times had changed and we would take the risk. Immanuel was to drive the Buick Skylark with Darleen and the three older children, and we would take the Chevrolet station wagon with the three younger children. Everything went smoothly until the second day of the trip when we stopped at a hot dog stand in a small town in Arkansas.

"Our family was served at the window immediately, but Immanuel and Darleen were intentionally ignored. We decided to leave, and drove the station wagon out onto the highway where we waited for the other car. Looking back, we noticed that there was a riot occurring and the Skylark was blocked in, surrounded with teenagers' sports cars, and Immanuel's only way out was to drive straight forward into a deep ditch. I started to walk back to see what the trouble was, although I knew very well that it was a racial problem. In the meantime, a plain-clothes man quelled the disturbance, had the cars cleared away, and Immanuel drove out to the highway to join us. I asked Immanuel if he had been afraid, and he answered, 'I knew God was with us.'

"When I asked the children what they thought about the disturbance, I realized that they did not sense that there was any connection to racial prejudice. Our eleven-year-old daughter said, 'I thought those teenagers were just being naughty.'

"The next day was Easter Sunday and we all attended church services in Hot Springs, Arkansas, where we were greeted politely. We proceeded on to New Orleans and were warmly welcomed at a motel that had only one room available. Eight had to sleep on the floor. The kids loved it.

"On the return trip, we stopped overnight at a motel in a small city in Arkansas, and wanting to be honest, I told the motel owner that we had a black man in our group. 'Don't tell me about it!' he retorted. Since it was late, we stayed that night, but the next morning we found all four of the tires on the Skylark had been slashed. We bought two new tires at $20.00 apiece, the other two were repaired, and we were on our way toward Memphis, Tennessee by 10:00 A.M. In Memphis we stopped to see the Martin Luther King Memorial where Dr. King had been assassinated on the second-floor balcony of the Lorraine Hotel on the fourth of April of previous year."

Now thirty years later his continued good health depended upon Al's willingness to admit his finer qualities, his admirable traits. As the analysis reported, it is easy for others to see the value of the life Al has lived, more difficult for the man himself.

We see that it is time for this one to begin to face both the enjoyable, pleasurable, commendable in the self as well as the undesirable, ridiculing, and despicable parts of the self. It would be of great benefit for this one to become attached to truth and to strive to be honest. This one has always valued honesty very highly, and in some ways can be truthful but this one does not know how to be truthful with the self. Would suggest that this one learn how.

Emotionally Al had established a pattern that brought an ease in expression. It required no investigation and for the most part his emotions were taken for granted. This is a common condition as people enter their elderly years. Those who rely heavily upon habitual ways of thinking and feeling, find their mental capacities and physical body rapidly aging. The initial cause of this is forgetting or in refusing to continue to learn. Continuing to learn throughout your life is the stimulus for creative energies that flow through mind and body, replenishing themselves each time we create, each time we give to others, each time we enhance someone else's life. By coming to terms with his ego-centered habits, Al would free himself of emotional restriction:

...We see that emotionally this one becomes stagnant in what this one would identify as approval or rejection. We see that in reality however this is a way for this one to deny his own standards of

accomplishment, his own code of ethics, his own ideas of morality. It is much easier for this one to both live up to as well as fail to live up to these codes of standards as long as this one believes they belong to someone else and not him. Would suggest to this one however that this one's thinking creates the self. It is the identity of the self and therefore whatever code of ethics of standards that this one has entertained, even when this one has tried to put them off on someone else, they are his own. Whatever this one has lived up to this one has earned, this one has made a part of self and will have the benefit of. Whatever this one has not adhered to, this one has not fed the self and does not have this to draw upon. This is the honesty spoken of...

Al's tendency to try to live up to others' expectations, and his desire to win others' acceptance was a smokescreen for how he was living his life. He used these ideas to rob himself of responsibility for how he was thinking. It was not others who forced him to be a certain way, it was Al who was for whatever reason forcing himself to be. The thing was, who Al had become was in large part heroic and admirable. He just needed to admit it.

The analysis went on to describe what these attitudes had produced in the body:

We see because of this in the physical body there is great difficulty in utilizing the senses fully. We see that there is a significant drop in the electrochemical movement to the auditory system and to the visual system. We see that in large part this is due to the denial of the emotions that have been spoken of and this one pulling back and away from life experiences. In order for the body to change this one will need to find a renewed willingness to look and see, to hear and listen, in the experiences.

While not to continue in the same comfortable path that this one has had for many years. We see it also greatly affects the body in terms of its nourishment. We see that although this one does give the body a wide variety of foods and for the most part an adequate amount, the body itself does not utilize it. The food substances are not broken down and there are not the necessary vitamins, minerals, and amino acids for this body to carry on all of its functions appropriately. There could be some benefit derived from fruit and vegetable juices taken daily. If these could be fresh, they will work much better for the body, particularly those of root crops such as beets. Turnips would also be a benefit for the body. Carrots, ginseng root would be useful to this body. Would suggest the use of coriander and peppers, more shellfish would be of use as well.

There is some sluggishness within the liver, and also the small intestines. The condition of the liver would be somewhat aided by a diet that would have less oil. This would include oily vegetables as avocados, as well as those high in animal fat. We see that for the most part the heart muscle is strong. We see some weakening of the valve in the atrium as there has been some pressure in the pulmonary artery. There is a need for more exercising of the tidal volume capacity of the lungs. Breathing exercises at least twice a day would be of help to the lungs and heart. There is the beginning of some breakdown in the connective tissue. This is in response to the long standing thinking that has already been described that this one has held onto and yet it is not really what this one desires. We see there would be a benefit for this body to be touched more often, it would stimulate the energy flows and it would cause a kind of awakening or resiliency in the cellular tissue which would be very helpful to the energy flows in this body. (4-17-93-BGC-a)

A physical area Al wanted to know about, a common concern for aging males in the United States, was the prostate gland. The analysis returned with the following:

There is swelling here and some dead tissue that has built up in this area. There is potential for malignancy in this area. In addition to what has already been given, would suggest that in this one's overlooking or denial of the emotions there are a very definite set of emotional patterns that this one established years ago. The ones that are relevant to this area as to the deadening, revolve around a resentment of someone in this one's mind that this one blames for keeping this one from choosing what he wanted, what he himself desired. It would be of benefit to explore this and to come to terms with it. This would cause some expansion in terms of thinking, but it would also stop feeding the disorder in this area. (4-17-93)

Al responded to this immediately. He had a good idea who and what the report was talking about from his past and he was determined to change his present. "As suggested in the analysis, I began to fulfill my here-to-fore squelched desires, and found that I had many capabilities that just needed freedom of expression. A load was lifted from my shoulders as I gave of myself and discovered that I had a lot of knowledge to offer to others." Retired from his business, Al is actively involved in his community. He volunteers time to lead discussion groups with men incarcerated for drug offenses. He teaches a Sunday School class of young people at the church he and his wife have attended for years. A lecturer and writer, he teaches continuing adult education classes and the SOM course in Chicago. He is a devoted husband, father, and grandfather.

Perhaps this story about Al's relationship with a Vietnamese family describes the kind of man Al is best. For he is the kind of person we all aspire to be. An independent septuagenarian, possessed of a good mind and sound body. One who is living a full life of meaning and substance.

"It was a Saturday afternoon on June 27th, 1975, at Mitchell Field Airport in Milwaukee, Wisconsin. As members of the St. Mary's Lutheran Church liaison team, my wife and I welcomed two Vietnamese families; we were to help them establish a new life in America. We met 12 Vietnamese men, women, and children who were wearing name tags so we could identify them. Each family had one suitcase and shared one cardboard box, their entire worldly possessions. Both families had escaped from their war-torn country with only one hour's notice, and were transported to Guam by boat. From there they were transferred to a refugee camp in Ft. Smith, Arkansas, where they were detained until a person or group could be found to sponsor them.

"The Nguyen family included parents, Toan and Tam, and three small children, a daughter Ha, and two sons, Bac and baby Chanh. With them were Toan's two adult single sisters, Lan Anh and Togiang. The Tran family consisted of Choung, the father, Thuy, his wife, two daughters, Tu Quynh 12, Van Anh 10, and an 8 year-old son, Chan.

"St. Mary's Lutheran Church, as sponsors, had already rented and furnished an apartment for each family and found employment for the men. Toan Nguyen had been an officer in the South Vietnamese Navy. Choung Tran was South Vietnam President Thieu's chief palace engineer and confidant. Thuy had been a grade school teacher. We kept almost daily contact with both families, assisting then with their English, filling out papers, teaching them to drive, taking their children to the doctor and dentist, and helping them with their daily problems. They were very responsive, and quickly became independent.

"Although the Vietnamese were Buddhists, they were anxious to become acquainted with the Christian Bible and our church. It was not long before they asked to participate in the Lord's Supper. I relayed their request to Pastor Pedersen who replied, "Everyone is welcome, invite them to come forward."

"In November of 1976, Lan Anh Nguyen married Huynh Son, a Vietnamese man she had met at Ft. Smith. My wife Elga and I were pleased when they requested that the wedding ceremony be held in our church, and asked us to serve as 'parents of the bride.' A year later we were asked to give away Lan Anh's sister Togiang in marriage.

"Another church in our city sponsored a Vietnamese family with four teenage daughters. The parents were orchard workers and none of the family knew English. At their welcoming party it was obvious that there was no friendship between our refugee families and the newcomers. Noticing this, we asked Toan Nyugen to talk to his countrymen and translate for them so they would feel more welcome. He wanted nothing to do with them – hey were 'uneducated orchard laborers.' I thought, 'a regular Vietnamese caste system.' Toan finally did consent to talk with them, but only for this event. We never heard what happened to this family.

"Choung Tran died of kidney failure in 1987. Before his death, his children asked if our church would give their father a Christian burial. 'Of course!' I said, 'If they don't I will have to leave the church.' When death came, a Christian funeral service was held at our church. The service was attended by members of our congregation and the Kenosha-Racine-Milwaukee area Vietnamese community. The following month we were invited to an outdoor Buddhist memorial service in Milwaukee.

"By 1993, Van Anh, now 28, had fallen in love with Mike, a fellow student at Marquette Dental School in Milwaukee. Her mother, Thuy, protested the engagement, 'we just do not mix races!' she exclaimed. 'I will not speak to them if they get married.' However it was not long before she changed her attitude, accepted Mike into the family, and gave the marriage her blessing, and the wedding was held in a Lutheran Church in Milwaukee. Since Van Anh's father had died, her uncle, a physician who had settled in Texas, sponsored the wedding and reception for 200 guests.

"In *Matthew, Chapter* 22 v. 37-40 Jesus says, 'You shall love the

Lord, your God, with all your heart, with all your soul, with all your mind. This is the greatest and the first commandment. The second is like it: you shall love your neighbor as yourself.' Almost everyone knows that they are happiest when they give love to others, and it is so simple and easy to do. We all respond to love, and it costs nothing to give. The church is an excellent place to reach out to others. In the above story the whole congregation (although there were a few grumblers) welcomed the Vietnamese into their circle and the Vietnamese responded with love."

In 1996, Al requested another Intuitive Health Analysis to aid in his spiritual progress, which is considerable. Al is a prime example that learning, growth, and change occurs when the mind is ready. It need not be impaired or limited in any way by the body. Nor do we ever outgrow our desire and capacity to learn.   What Al learned about himself in this analysis is good advice for anyone entering the years of wisdom.

We see that this one is very hard on the Self. We see that there are ideas that this one has formed that are firm in this one's mind concerning ideals and values that this one aspires to live up to. We see however, that in the choices that this one makes this one does not always abide by what this one believes to be true and correct. We see as a result of this, this one becomes very critical, very condemning, very self-deprecating.

Would suggest to this one that when this one views a difference between what this one believes or values and what this one actually practices, that simply berating the Self does not cause this change. Would suggest that at those times this one formulate very clear goals concerning what this one wants to build, what this one wants to develop, what this one wants to accomplish. Would suggest that these goals be reasonable such that this one can move toward them and accomplish them. For we see that there are times when this one does set goals that are so far out of reach, as this one sees it, that this one simply gives up and then repeats the cycle of self criticism.

It would be suggested as well that this one appreciate the self for what this one has accomplished and the ways that this one has lived up to the values of the Self. We see that this one has difficulty giving the Self credit for this and therefore, holds back in giving what this one has to give in this regard.

We see that within the emotional system that this one dwells upon negative emotions particularly, those from the past that this one has not resolved. It would be suggested that this one learn how to forgive the Self and others for mistakes and errors. Following the suggestions that have been related in regard to setting goals will aid in this regard as well.

We see within the physical body there is a stiffening that is occurring in the joint areas and the muscular system; deep muscle massage would be recommended, exercise that moves the joint areas would be recommended, relaxing mentally, emotionally and physically would be recommended.

We see that there is an irregular heartbeat. We see that much of this is brought upon by this one's dwelling upon emotions from the past. Suggestions have been given in that regard. The intake of hawthorn or coenzyme Q-10 could be of some benefit.

There is some enlargement in the prostate, would suggest the intake of saw palmetto. Would suggest that this one drink more water and chew the food more thoroughly in order to assimilate its nutrients. This is all.

Q: Is additional zinc of any value here in the area of the prostate? *This could be of benefit.*

Q: What would be the easiest way for this one to build new understandings, permanent understandings?
The first step lies in this one evaluating the understandings that have already been built and causing the Self to give of these and from these on a regular basis. This will aid in stimulating this one's awareness of what is already present within the Self...This one needs to move his own attention from what is wrong with the Self to what this one has gained and accomplished. (2-17-96-LJC-M)

Al credits his health analysis as a revealing and motivating force in this new stage of his life. It has helped him to have a focus for his learning, a clearer purpose for his existence. Acting on the suggestions, particularly to aid others has given him a future. The more he teaches and encourages those younger than himself, the more he becomes invested in their growth and learning. This returns back to him, replenishing his desire to continue learning.

Al is in the mainstream of life and anyone who has the great honor of knowing him is very glad. His love of others is what fuels his mind and body. His willingness to learn something new is an inspiration to people of all ages and a lesson for those who have stopped learning too soon. The wisdom that pours from his life experience is a bounty for us all.

Life for Al is how it can be for anyone reaching for that centenarian mark. "I now awake in the morning with joy, anxious to meet the challenges of each new day."

"Last scene of all"

"In the summer of 1989 my dad had been complaining of being tired and was also constipated much of the time," says Ernie Padilla. The story of him and his father is both heart-warming and heart-breaking. Touching in the ways it speaks to all of us who sooner or later must say goodbye to those we have loved so very much.

"On New Year's of 1990 my dad was complaining of not feeling very well. He did not care much for doctors and put off going to one for a long time. The first doctor he visited in Castle Rock (Colorado) where he lived did not catch the condition he was ailing of. My father's brother, Dave finally had him go to his doctor because the condition was worsening. It was then that the doctor was suspicious of cancer."

Shortly thereafter Ernest Sr. was diagnosed with colon cancer. In May, doctors at the University of Colorado operated on him. "When they operated, they discovered the cancer was everywhere including the lymph nodes. They immediately closed him up. The doctors told my Aunt Sharon that dad had about three to six months to live."

Even with this prognosis, physicians began chemotherapy and radiation treatments and Ernest Sr. became subject to the type of "cancer treatment" Western medicine offers. "My dad experienced vomiting, craving certain foods, and yet he had trouble eating. He became thinner and thinner, shriveling up." He was dying before Ernie's eyes. "We had a family reunion in the month of July. By then dad was in a wheelchair. Many relatives got to see him and held onto him tight."

"In August, my dad gave up the battle, dying on August 8, 1990. He was only fifty years old."

"I remember my Dad telling me he had cancer.
"At first I couldn't believe it. I thought of his history, his anger, blaming others. I loved my dad. I cared and wanted to help him.

"My studies at the School of Metaphysics included wholistic health. I knew why dad had cancer, but my knowing this did not ease his pain." Using what he had learned about healing did. Ernie projected healing energy to his dad almost daily. Others who wanted to help gave their time and energy to offset the ravages of the disease and the treatment.

When the doctors wanted to give his dad a new experimental drug on top of the chemotherapy he'd already endured, Ernie decided it was time to set aside any fear on his part of what his dad might think and let him know about intuitively-accessed health information. Ernie wanted his dad to know that something existed that could help him help himself. "I had a tool to help him if he wanted to change. This tool was an Intuitive Health Analysis from the School of Metaphysics which had been researching and studying cancer and the thoughts that create this. I finally talked to him about the health analysis. He agreed to receive one."

What the analysis reported affected Ernest Sr. in ways Ernie never imagined. It opened his dad's eyes to truths he had ignored throughout his life. It filled in missing pieces for Ernie concerning why his dad had done some of the things he did. It resolved old misunderstandings, replacing them with acceptance and love, offering closure for both father and son.

We see this one spends too much time in this one's thoughts justifying the acts and choices this one has made. We see that there is a need for this one to learn to make choices, to expect them to be worthy and functional, and to move on to the next subject or activity in the life.

There is a need for this one to stop worrying about whether the choices were right or wrong. If this one was wrong, this one can correct it when this one sees that it is wrong. There is a need for this one to do this in order to see that there is not a need to justify the choices either. We see that if this one was able to be more conscious and intentional and purposeful about thinking out the decisions that this one has to make, rather than making snap judgements or functioning from the emotions, this one would be more sure of the self in this regard and would trust the self more in making the choices. Therefore (he) would not have to justify them so much in the thinking.

This takes up a lot of time, this justifying, this one could be using the mind for something else. This one could be learning or enjoying. This is a habit, this one needs to see it as a habit, just as tangible as a physical habit and to change it.

Ernie could remember from his childhood experience extreme examples of what his dad might now be trying to come to terms with. Ernest Sr.'s uncontrolled thoughts often bred emotional outbursts that ended in physical violence. "My dad was the kind of guy who demanded a lot of respect. He was going to get it from you one way or another. I know that there was a time when I was about fourteen, some friends of mine and I were in the garage. My dad wanted me to do something and I smarted off to him. I was bending over picking something up and he walked over and kicked me in the face in front of all my friends. That's an example of something he would do, more out of fear.

"There were times we'd be in the car. He and mom would be arguing and he always had to be right. Even to the point to where he might hit my mom. Then my mom would start crying and say 'I can't believe you hit me.' He would say, 'I didn't hit you.' He'd look back at us kids and say, 'Did I hit her?' And we're all saying, 'No, no, no,' out of fear of retribution. These are the habits he had." Incapacitated by illness, Ernest Sr. was now facing his own judgments of the kind of life he had lived, seeking peace for the choices he had made.

What most helped Ernie to understand his father were the following insights:

We see that it would be very beneficial for this one to be giving attention to what this one has learned about the spirituality and the religion this one has learned throughout this one's life.

It would be beneficial for this one to ask the self now the kinds of questions this one asked the self and mostly to other people around the self, authority figures around the self in this one's teenage years and older childhood years. This one has accumulated some wisdom and there is a need for this one to ask the self those questions and to think about them in order for this one to hear the answers that this one has accumulated over time. Either that or to put the self around teenagers, around older children in a kind of capacity where this one can then ask the self questions and would have to come up with answers to similar questions that this one asks about religion and about life in the earlier years.

"After listening to this I knew there was a certain way of thinking that dad had where he was living a con. The con was really on himself.

"I know my grandmother was very spiritual. She was the matriarch of the family and he was very close to her. I know there was a part of him that had spiritual roots, and desires. But there was a certain standard of living physically that he desired. His thoughts and attitudes and values I know were not important to the kinds of women he coupled with after the divorce (from Ernie's mother).

As close as Ernest Sr. was to his mother he was estranged from his father. Ernie knew very little about him since he died when Ernie was young. "When my grandfather died he gave me a violin. I asked my dad what he received and dad said, 'I didn't expect nothing, my dad's never given me anything.' That was a shock to me. After a week or two, the violin my grandfather had given me was gone. To this day I don't know what happened to it, but I have ideas.

"I remember nobody in the family talked about my grandfather. It was an unspoken rule, no one says anything about him. It was like 'as long as you don't have anything good to say about someone then you don't talk about it.' My grandfather must have had some talents because as I played guitar and sang at my sister's wedding and everybody was saying, 'you're just like your grandfather, he sang and played guitar.' That's about the only good thing I heard about my grandfather. And one of the few things I ever learned about him. Now I know it was because dad would not tolerate even the mention of him."

The deep seated issues between Ernie's father and grandfather had festered for years in his dad. Whatever demons plagued his dad, they helped shape his dad's life and relations with his own family.

"I knew that he didn't completely express what was on his mind, what was important. He was living a different life than what he believed in. It was very apparent at the time he got his reading and his second wife could see much of it."

We see this one has a need to be aware of what has been learned throughout the life that would cause this one to realize the life has been worthwhile and that this one has made a great deal more progress in understanding (than) this one imagines or thinks the self is capable of. This one has already accomplished a great deal more within the life than this one ever thought the self capable of, but this one needs to see it. It needs to be seen because this one still has things to do.

"Many people looked up to my dad and respected him. He was an example for a lot of people.

"Dad was a lithographer for the government. He didn't talk about his work. I always thought he kept it secret from us, maybe he wasn't supposed to discuss it. I'll never know. He would repeatedly say, 'I don't bring my work home.' As far as I could tell I believed him.

"There was one day, I was probably about 12 or 13 years old. It was a school day and you were to go out to work with somebody. My dad let me and a couple of my friends go to see what he did. That was the only time that happened. It was then that I found out what a lithographer does."

This one does not even recognize the self is capable of doing things although this one will think that someone needs to do something about them. This one is capable of doing something about them, and needs to do this for this one's growth, satisfaction and feeling of well-being within the life.

We see that within the emotional system that this one feels a little bit betrayed and feels as though there has been a lack of action within the life to fulfill needs.

"My dad did feel betrayed by life because he felt the world did owe him something. Particularly since he had compromised himself. There were many ways he had been living that he didn't want to be doing, from getting married because my mother was pregnant to doing the work he was doing. Most of what was in his life did not reflect what he really wanted, or at least what he thought was going to be what he wanted. Life had betrayed him because it hadn't brought him the satisfaction he expected."

We see that this has not been true because this one did not realize what has been learned within the life and that this one does degrade

*the self and put the self down. This one has received within the life
what this one needed, just as this one continues to do so now. It
would change this one's life and change this one's thinking to
recognize what this one truly has learned. Would suggest to this one
to learn some type of public speaking or teaching. We see that
within the emotional system that this one feels somewhat lonely
even when this one is around people because this one is not giving
what this one could offer people from this one's experiences
therefore this one feels isolated.*

*We see that within the physical system that this one is having
difficulty processing information within the brain. In other words,
this one thinks slowly and does not fully put together concepts in the
present time. That is because of the present attitude of boredom. It
is also because this one is putting the self in positions of the need to
think because this one does not think enough in a creative or
intelligent manner.*

*There is difficulty in the reasoning processes and the neuron and
electrodes within the brain. We see that this could be corrected by
doing eye exercises, concentration exercises, and by verbalizing
this one's thoughts particularly the creative inventive thoughts this
one has.*

"Much of this disorientation was the result of the chemotherapy," Ernie
noted.

Even though knowledge is more widespread these days, people still
want to believe that the chemicals used in Western medicine do what they
are designed to do: kill cancer. They also want to believe that physicians
hold to the first Hippocratic tenet: First do no harm. The chemicals do
destroy cancer cells. They also target and kill healthy cells leaving the body
ravaged and severely weakened. Thus doctors, although they believe they
are justified, break the first commitment they make as a physician for in the
majority of cases chemotherapy inflicts unimaginable pain and radical
decline of health into death. And there have been enough experiments to
predict the few cases where it might be an answer.

Ernest Sr.'s analysis details the effects of disease and treatment upon
the brain and body. The greatest disruption is upon the ability to think
clearly. When the chemicals, noted as acids in the analysis, impair the
functioning of the brain and nervous system the reasoning capacity of the
mind is lessened.

What is notable about this analysis is how it is focused upon the immediate condition of the body. Unlike other analyses where benign or malignant tumors are described, this analysis addresses the other conditions as primary, those related to easing physical pain more than recovery which is an indication that the process of withdrawal (dying) has begun.

> *Within the physical system, there is tension along the spine. We see that there is a need for massage, particularly close to the spine. This one is experiencing calcium deposits along this area which need to be stimulated to dissolve. Massage would do this, so would ultrasound, so would ultraviolet rays.*
>
> *We see there is a need for nutmeg in the diet. Approximately one quarter of a teaspoon in a gelatin capsule. This needs to be taken daily for three or four months and this is to remove the release of waste from the reproductive organs. Therefore to promote the right hormones and vitality and to release waste that is producing something similar to stones.*
>
> *There is a need for the intake of acidophilus to help balance the digestion. This one has too much acid within the system at the present time. There is a need for more fruits and vegetables and nuts within the diet. There is a need for more physical rest. It would be beneficial for this one to use more honey in the diet rather than artificial sweeteners. This is all.*

Q: Not too long ago this one was operated on for colon cancer and at the present time has been diagnosed and has liver cancer and cancer of the lymph nodes. You will examine for this condition and relate.

> *We see that this one is having difficulty in the release of waste fluids from these areas. There is a need for more fluid intake into the system and to release this from these areas and to eliminate toxins within the fluids in these areas. We see that there is a need for this one to recognize that although there are counteractive measures within the body to heal the body, there is a need to cooperate in this one's thinking. There is a need to accept this one's own value. There is a need for this one to realize that in order to really complete the goals and the life that there is a need to express from the self what this one has learned in this period of time.*

The body has endured radical treatment, therefore most of the analysis centers on Ernest's need to cooperate with the measures already taken and to resolve the life with understanding. The analysis clearly places the power of life and death in Ernest's hands. In its personal counsel to him is revealed Truths that apply to us all.

> *We see that although this one has experienced some destruction within these areas, there is also healthy tissue within these areas. That is not to say that there are not difficulties, but that this one is quite capable of fulfilling what this one needs to give and fulfill what this one needs to do to have a sense of well being and yet a sense of health. Would suggest to this one that it is not the body that tells this one when to die or it is not the body that becomes diseased on its own (rather it is) the thinking, the goals, that determine whether this one is capable of producing health within the body or producing disease within the body. We see that there is not an active growth of cancer within these areas. There is a mass of tissues within these areas that has formed into a gel-like substance and has not been released from the body. There are also inactive cells in these areas that are abnormal cells. That is all.*

> Q: What is the mental cause that has produced the liver cancer?
> *The mental cause is based on this one's thinking that there is not anything very important to live for. That there is hurt and disappointment, that there has not been something more to the life than what there has been. We see this one has not blamed anyone else, that this one has felt very bad that this one has not accomplished more in the life.*

Ernie can readily see these patterns of thinking in his father. From the sacrifice of his religious principles to actively acting against what he believed to be right, he made parts of his life worthless by giving up, over and over again.

"My mom and dad got divorced when I was about 14. Part of what led up to the divorce was that we had an ice cream parlor called the Peppermint Shake. It was in a great location near the high school. We lived in a nice house. Dad was in partnership with my uncle and after about a year the business went bankrupt. That's when my mom started blaming him and that's when we were losing everything, the house and so forth.

"I think he still worked for the government after that. But I knew he always ended up being with these women who were very independent, strong, and wealthy. The women were already established, had their own houses, many were divorced.

"I know that living a certain lifestyle was important to my dad. He drove a Black Porsche. He would have driven a Corvette, but the insurance rates were ridiculous. He was the kind of guy who was tall, dark, and handsome. And he knew it. He had used it all his life to get the lifestyle he wanted." Now, as he faced death Ernest was discovering that the attainment of lifestyle is empty when appearance is your sole ambition in life. Overwhelmed by this realization, Ernie's dad couldn't see how his presence had affected others in ways that transcend what money can buy or how things look.

We see that it is oblivious to this one what this one has accomplished, of the lives that this one has touched. If this one would recognize the lives this one has touched, what this one has learned, and be more open and intentional about giving to people what this one wants to give to them then this one would not be able to produce the cancer within the liver.

Q: What's the mental attitude that has caused the cancer to manifest in the lymphatic system?
This was secondary and after cancer manifested within the liver, this was produced by the apathy that then took over in this one's thinking.

Q: The physicians that are tending to this one are suggesting a type of chemical therapy that is relatively new and experimental. Do you find this would be beneficial or detrimental to the cancer cells within this body?
Would suggest to this one that part of the consideration would be the health of the kidneys at the present time. Would suggest that there would be a need for this one to evaluate the thoughts and to make sure there is not guilt that this one is holding within the self. There is a need also to make sure physically that at the time it would be taken that the kidneys are physically working properly for one of the side effects of this experimentation is upon the kidneys. Would suggest to this one also that the main determination that would cause

the drug to work within the physical system would be this one's own expectations and acknowledgement of it. We see that it could be useful to this one if this one has a sense of hope or somewhere this one wants to go with the life. Would suggest to this one that if this one's will to live is not present, that the drug could cause a great deal of confusion, difficulty within coherency and some physical damage to the life as well.

Tentative, yet determined, Ernie brought a cassette recording of the analysis to his father. "I remember the afternoon so well sitting at the dinner table with my dad and my step-mom. He put the cassette in the player and began to listen. When he was finished listening to it with us he looked up at me and said, 'There is no way anyone could know those things about me.'

"For me, and I think my dad, this analysis opened up a new door for us. I talked with my Dad about the analysis. He knew the suggestions were accurate and he was momentarily 'in remission.'

"Even though he decided to give up rather than fight to recover, I knew I had mentally connected with him before he died. He now knew I was doing a great service by attending the School of Metaphysics; he knew firsthand the kind of work I was doing. His respect was important to me. And I needed to know that I had brought something valuable to my dad.

"Because of what I had learned about myself and the nature of man's consciousness in general, it was much easier for me to understand and act upon the suggestions for family members given in the analysis. To the question, "Are there any further suggestions for those surrounding this one, particularly the close family members?" the intuitive reporter responded:

Would suggest to these ones by giving attention to the body only these ones do themselves a disservice and do not open up their minds to receiving what this one has to give to them. Would suggest to these ones to reach with their mind and to the mind of this individual...although they are afraid that they might be hurt to open up their own thinking, to receive whatever this one has to say to them. Would suggest to these ones that what they might learn would be from their actions rather than from this one's words. It is very important to their learning and to their being able to communicate to this one and to having a sense of positiveness for there to be attention put on this one as an individual and not just a body. (5-15-90-CR-1)

In retrospect Ernie realizes just how valuable his dad's analysis was to him. Not only as a means to help his father, something to give to him, but as an education about ending physical life with peace, dignity, and compassion. "Initially I wanted to understand why dad had gotten cancer, and the analysis helped me to understand it. I connected with dad before he died in ways we had never experienced before. I was learning about death firsthand. The relatives kept holding onto him as long as they could, keeping my dad here, in the physical world. To some degree I came to peace with his death because I had given him something. And he had received it.

"Dad never shared this knowledge (in the intuitive analysis) with other relatives and I respected that. Yet I knew without doubt that what I had brought to him was a new insight into himself that I believe in some ways eased his passing.

"I remember a week before my Dad died. My relatives were asking him who gave the best massages, one of his analysis' major suggestions for his physical body. They wanted to know, for some reason. Everyone in the family massaged him while he was diseased."

Ernie stops, reflective. A warm glow rises in his countenance. It is easy to tell that the final memory of his dad is one that brings him joy.

"I'll always remember his reply, 'My son Ernie gives the best foot massages'."

How we respond to the end of life is determined by how we live life.
For many it is more difficult to witness another's passing than to face their own. Pam Blosser is well acquainted with the depth of content and the multiplicity of applications in Intuitive Health Analyses. She gained personal experience with one of these when her mother died in early 1997.

Pam knew her mother was ill. A few years earlier her mother had a life-threatening condition. Pam encouraged her to receive an intuitive analysis, which she did. Midst the different suggestions, Pam's mom chose surgery from which she recovered.

When Pam's mother was diagnosed with bone cancer, she was not expected to live long. She did not request another analysis, nor did Pam offer. This time the Intuitive Health Analysis would be not for the one dying but for the one who would continue to live. Pam's choice to have a health analysis on herself at this time gave her the perspective she needed for her own peace of mind and the intuitive insight she wanted for what she could then bring to her mother in her last earthly days.

Pam's story paints a picture of deepening compassion and realizations well-earned during one of the most poignant moments in anyone's life. What she learned teaches us something about saying goodbye. Beyond that, how she came to the understandings she gained teaches us a great deal about saying hello to life, to love, to new parts of ourselves.

"I had been to visit my mother shortly after her diagnosis. When I returned home I tried to get right back into the day-to-day duties of my life. What I found was activities or people's words and actions would be the stimulus to open the floodgates of my emotions. I seemed to be swept away in the current of my own swirling feelings, starting to cry for no apparent reason. Other times the tides of my reactions ebbed and flowed from apathy, "I don't care," to anger. What was the thought that precipitated these outbursts? How could I quiet the roar of emotion to hear my thoughts?

"After about four days the torrents still persisted. I needed and wanted help. I wanted to be buoyed up to a renewal of peace. I wanted a lifeline to truth. I knew I could get both from an Intuitive Health Analysis and that's what I decided to do.

"The analysis began..."

> *We see anxiety within this one. We see that in many regards this one is not satisfied with the self and with the life and there are many stimuli that bring this to this one's attention. When these are brought to this one's attention this one becomes engrossed in anxiety or worry or condemnation rather than coming to a point of understanding, release and change.*

"I could identify the anxiety the reading described. There were changes professionally that were going on. There were changes going on in my physical body that I was very much aware of and then there was the change of my mother dying."

"My life was a busy one. I love what I do but sometimes I have trouble keeping up with all of it. Sometimes it seems everywhere I looked, unfinished projects, books half read, unanswered mail and other miscellaneous clutter were screaming at me for attention and a response. How could I reply with a sense of peace and perspective? My answer was, more often than not, one of anxiety."

Would suggest to this one that there is need for this one to embrace change. We see that this one has intellectual concepts regarding this but in regards to actually causing this and loving this, this one has great difficulty with this. We see that much of what is occurring at the present time is that there are many external circumstances in this one's existence that are changing and this one has great difficulty accepting this, appreciating this, and using this for her own growth and her own expansion.

"I was aware of the steps to causing change and there had been progress in regard to responding to needs for growth and maturity. But exercising this process as a daily part of my consciousness was not yet fully present. I hadn't yet learned how to transform and mature my consciousness without anxiety. It was habitual for me to become anxious about having the time, energy and ability to do all the things I wanted to do and keep everything in perspective.

"In regards to my mother's condition, I was anxious about how I could leave my busy life to be with her the last days of her life. I was anxious about my father and his ability and strength to take care of her. I was aware of this anxiety. There were two other factors of anxiety I wasn't aware of that were revealed in the reading."

One is that this one fears that her own hidden resentments have the probability of producing this kind of condition within herself.

"I had observed anger in my mother. I was conscious of anger within myself. I had witnessed the high standards that my mother had with herself and other people and the judgments she made. I was aware of the same thing within myself. The anger and condemnation I had experienced in my life left me a prime candidate for cancer. I knew that many of my thoughts were like my mother's. My mother dying of cancer was coming very close to home to the possibility of my dying of cancer. The reality of this thought scared me."

The second is that this one harbors regrets about her own life and this one has not ever really faced the mortality of the self. This experience is bringing to her attention a deeper awareness of her own mortality.

"For the first time in my life I was coming to face my own mortality. This reality was not just a possibility that I might die of cancer but the inevitable fact that I was going to die. Someday I would not be here in this physical form that I existed in today. This was the more universal and essential factor needing to be responded to and embraced.

"I had told myself for years I was not afraid of death. As a young girl I had read a book about life after death and an existence beyond the physical that I believed true and had brought me comfort as well as a false sense of security. Death had been a remote experience, one that I heard about or saw enacted on television. I knew at the time of death the consciousness of the individual leaves the body but the actual process of dying and preparation for death was a mystery to me. I hadn't been around anyone who was dying nor witnessed death much less the death of a loved one. Philosophically I had said, 'My parents are going to die someday' but I had yet to face the reality of this truth where I could taste the realness of death that I was now tasting. Yet this taste, at first bitter in my mouth, became sweet in my stomach as I cared for my mother and witnessed the dying process.

"In asking about how to help my mother with her transition the analysis suggested"

This one can give love to this other. This one can share the knowledge this one has about knowledge that is beyond the physical. This one can pray with this other. It would be suggested that this one draw upon the spiritual education that this one has in examining what this one can offer to this other that she does not know.

"These brought a great sense of comfort and peace for there was a lot I could offer my mother in her transition. She believed in a heaven and an afterlife and had read about life after death so I know she had some idea about the soul separating from the physical body. Because she identified with the physical body she had no idea how to release her soul from her physical entrapment. This was where I could help her.

"There was about a two week period between times of staying with my mother. Her health had deteriorated substantially in that time. She was still lucid to some extent. She was on morphine to kill the pain. Her mental faculties were still intact. She was moving in and out of the inner levels and becoming more weakened as she approached death. Her body had diminished. She was eating and drinking less which I had learned is part of the dying process. Since it was getting more difficult for her to talk, she didn't say much. I knew I needed to talk to her and I wanted to talk to her.

"She kept repeating 'I don't understand...' and her voice would trail off before she finished her sentence. Finally she was able to get the whole sentence out. It was, 'I don't understand how I got myself into this mess.' She didn't understand how she could have lived a healthy life, taken good care of herself, and tried to be a good person and now be in such pain at the end. As long as I could remember, my mother had eaten healthily, exercised, and taken good care of herself. She and my father prided themselves in the fact that they had not been on a lot of medication. I don't remember her being sick very often. She had also tried to be a good person. She had high morals and had taught us to live by these as well.

"I told her I knew it was hard to understand, when she had tried to live a good life, why she should be having so much pain at the end but that she would understand very soon. I told her there would be a light that she could go to and there would be those who had passed on before her that would be waiting to greet and help her: brothers Jerry and Sam, her parents, her friend Lawana, and the angels. It would be peaceful and she would have the answers to her questions. In fact, she would understand many things about her life. She listened and then whispered faintly but with affirmation, 'Yes.'

"Yes, life continues in other forms and on other planes. Yes, truth does bring peace. Yes, there is an order behind what seems to be chaos in this world. Yes, love is eternal. And then we prayed together.

"Her attention continued to move in and out from her body to the inner levels of consciousness. I communicated with her through my thoughts, my touch and my words. With the help of the hospice people who came to the house and the information they had brought for us to read, through caring for my mother, I gained a greater understanding of the dying process. Yes, even though there can be pain, death in and of itself is a gentle transition. And yes, there is a beauty to dying. I definitely felt blessed that

I could be there for both my parents and witness my mother's passing.

"During the last days of my mother's life and the days after her death as we made all the arrangements for the funeral, I had very little attention on my own needs. My attention was given to my mother's needs and my father's needs. I was willing to do whatever it took to respond and give to the present moment. I wanted to aid my mother in her transition. I wanted to ease my father's grief, if possible, and help with all the arrangements. By helping my mother to be as comfortable as possible, giving her my love in the last moments of her life, and witnessing her passage from the physical into the spiritual realm, there was an inner transformation that I received that was directly related to what was in this health analysis.

"Since that time, I have my moments of anxiety but not to the extent that I had before. I think it was because in this time I was not anxious about myself. I was not anxious about what needed to be taken care of at my work. I needed to be where I was and doing what I was doing and that was the most important thing. The rest would take care of itself. I would be able to take care of it when I returned. I released my anxiety about what other things I needed to be getting done that I couldn't do. I think that kind of giving brought me a great amount of transformation and change and helped me to understand how to give my attention to something fully.

"My mother's disease was the result of some creative thinking that had gone awry. Everybody has creativity. When that creative energy is used to produce anger, anxiety, resentment, or fear we're still using our precious creative energy yet it's not contributing to anything of worth.

"This was an idea that I began to receive and process in my thinking. Anxiety wasn't going to bring me anything except possibly the illness that I observed my mother having. I had creative energy and I would get mileage out of it by disregarding my fears, doubts, and anxieties and giving my attention to my desires, goals, standards, ideals, and dreams. Another line from the analysis gave me greater insight about directing my mind. It was this"

> *The cause for the out-of-control, as this one views it, is this one allowing the attention to wander. (3-18-97-LJC-7)*

"I recognized that the out of control was in my control. I did have control of my thoughts and I could cause my attention to be where I wanted it to be. I could cause it to be on creating something that would span the test of time, that would contribute to the evolution of humanity. By controlling my thinking, my influence is what I truly want it to be. It's one that is ongoing and transformative not only for myself and for those around me but also for those who are at a distance in time and space. How I choose to direct my thinking has a myriad of repercussions on humanity and the maturation and growth of civilization. I am always in control of my attention.

"I began to see life as the expression of the creative urge and also how attention is used. In witnessing the last days of my mother's life, I saw how simple life could be. Reducing our existence to life and death strips away a lot of things that once were thought important. You see what seemed monumental to not really amount to a hill of beans. What does become important is how and what you create now, how and what you give to and receive from in the present moment, now.

"All you have is the present moment. What you do with it creates eternity."

The Five Stages of Living

Where did the body that you had when you were fourteen go?
What happened to it? Did it disappear into thin air? Does it still exist in your now fifteen or thirty or seventy-year-old body?

Everything in nature is resurrection.

In modern society we tend to lose sight of this Universal Truth. In nature, uninterrupted by man's desire and will, resurrection is abundant. Nestled deep in the earth under blankets of snow rests the acorn which will sprout and mature in springtime, flourish and produce offspring throughout the summer's warmth, then release its young during the technicolor foliage of autumn. All so the cycle of birth, life, death, and resurrection can be fulfilled. From the acorn to the mighty oak to the acorn the cycle brings resurrection. The dead trees of winter seem to be reborn each spring. And indeed they are.

Man is also subject to these cycles of existence. Being farther along in the evolutionary process, he possesses a creative power and volition unique to his species. "The paragon of animals," Shakespeare called him. In fact Shakespeare's intuitive insight into the reality and the promise of the human species is brilliant:

"What a piece of work is man!
How noble in reason! how infinite in faculty!
in form, in moving, how express and admirable!
in action how like an angel!
in apprehension how like a god!
the beauty of the world!
the paragon of animals!"
Hamlet (1601) act 2, sc. 2, 1.(316)

To understand this image of man is to live in harmony with the Universal Laws. Embracing the ebb and flow of life while exercising your capacity to create through thought.

However, this is often not our reality. Civilization in the 1900's has increasingly moved man away from contact with nature, the earth, the elements, toward meccas of his own design. Consider the dilemma. If your entire life is spent living in manmade houses, driving manmade cars on manmade concrete roads, working in manmade buildings filled with artificially cooled or heated air, eating processed foods and watching fictionalized accounts of human experience, contact with the rest of creation is minimal. In a manmade world, when our bodies are too hot we make the environment cool or we place a manmade lake where once there was a hill so we can take a refreshing swim. When we want a lawn in the middle of a concrete jungle created by man we transplant one, watering it when it doesn't rain, fertilizing it because no animals are present to provide it. When we want milk we go to a building where we purchase a waxed cardboard container filled with white liquid that, to protect our health, has been heated to kill bacteria then chemicals added to restore the vitamins lost in the process. When we miss someone who is far away we pick up a telephone receiver, push some buttons, and within seconds we hear the voice we long for as if the person was sitting next to us. As a society we can cause change in our environment very easily. And we do. We can do no less; man's innate urge is to create.

The challenge is to change in alignment with nature, otherwise self-indulgence is our undoing.

Consider the challenges of man as a creator.– Countless children without parents whether the consequence of divorce or war or government subsidy. Billions of tons of unusable trash no one knows what to do with, remnants from things we feel we must have in our life. Air we can't breathe, water we don't dare drink, and soil that won't produce anything usable. Animals and produce filled with so many chemicals, from antibiotics to insecticides, that whether consumption is healthy becomes debatable. Artificial life created by connecting the body to machines that fill the lungs with air and pump nourishment into the bloodstream. The lesson is clear: we are accountable for what we bring into existence.

The heights and pitfalls of man playing God have been the subject of philosophical discussion for centuries. With today's technology we must be willing to move beyond debate into the arena of purposeful action. What better way to do so than to once again become students of nature. To observe the workings of nature without thought of controlling it in some way. Quite a challenge for a species enthralled by its ability to press buttons and make something happen.

The insatiable lust for instant gratification causes most if not all the ills of the world be they personal disease or societal disorder. Most governments seek to control it, either through the ideals of equality among people found in a republic or the equality of property ownership in communism. Every religion on earth teaches the perils of lust. Lust is one of the seven mortal sins in Catholicism and in Hinduism lust is one of the three gates to self-destructive hell. Lust heats the heart and mind, generating a fervor of madness illustrated in shocking imagery by a man named Angulimala.

For almost 3000 years generation after generation his story has been told. It is said he was a madman. Because society had not treated him well he took a vow that he would kill one thousand people as his revenge. From every person killed he took a finger and made a rosary that he wore around his neck.

The man was called Angulimala, the man with a rosary of fingers.

He had killed nine hundred and ninety-nine people. Wherever he traveled people would stop. It became difficult for him to find that last man and only one more man was needed to fulfill his vow.

Buddha was approaching a forest, and people came to him from the villages saying, "Don't go! Angulimala is there, that mad murderer! He doesn't think about what he is doing, he just kills. He will not think of the fact that you are a Buddha. Go another way..."

But Buddha replied, "If I don't go, then who will go? He is a man, he needs me. I must go. Either he will kill me or I will kill him."

Buddha went. Even his closest disciples lagged behind.

When Buddha approached the hill where Angulimala was sitting on a rock there was no one behind him. He was alone.

Angulimala looked at this innocent man, childlike, so beautiful that even he, a murderer, felt compassion for him. He thought, "this man seems absolutely unaware that I am here. Nobody comes along this path. It is not good to kill this man. I'll leave him, I can find someone else to fulfill my vow."

He shouted to Buddha, "Go back! Stop there now and go back. Don't move another step. I am Angulimala. These are nine hundred and ninety-nine fingers here and I need only one more. Even if my mother comes I will kill her to fulfill my vow! So don't come near. I am dangerous!

"I am not a believer in religion," he continued. "You may be a monk, or a great saint, I don't care. Your finger is as good as anybody else's. Stop or I will kill you."

Buddha kept coming. Angulimala thought, Either this man is deaf or he is mad. "Stop I say!"

Buddha said, "I stopped long ago. I am not moving Angulimala, you are moving. There is no goal for me. And when there is no motivation, how can movement happen? You are moving, and I say to you, you stop!"

Angulimala laughed, "You are really a fool or you are mad. I don't know what manner of man you are."

Buddha came closer. "I have heard that you need one more finger. As far as this body is concerned, my goal is achieved, this body is useless. You can use it, your vow can be fulfilled—cut off my finger and cut off my head. I have come on purpose, because this is the last chance for my body to be used in some way."

Angulimala said, "I thought I was the madman here. Don't try to be clever, because I can still kill you."

Buddha said, "Before you kill me, do one thing. Just the wish of a dying man. Cut off a branch of this tree." Angulimala hit his sword against the tree and a big branch fell down.

Then Buddha said, "Just one thing more: join it again to the tree."

Angulimala said, "Now I know perfectly that you are mad. I can cut but I cannot join."

Then Buddha laughed, "When you can only destroy and cannot create you should not destroy. Destruction can be done by children, there is no bravery in it. This branch can be cut by a child; but to join it a Master is needed. And if you cannot even join back a branch to the tree, what about human heads? Have you ever thought about that?"

Angulimala closed his eyes and he said, "Lead me on that path." And it is said that in that single moment he became enlightened.

Eventually every person must master his own Self, facing his madness, his demon, his insatiable lust. Only by doing so are we willing to learn from the changes we bring about through our desires. Only by so doing can we convert the self-indulgent society into a spiritually advanced one. A civilization comprised of visionaries whose thoughts and actions are based, as in several American Indian philosophies, upon their effects seven generations from now.

The true challenge of man as a creator lies not in his ability to change things outside of himself, but rather in his capacity to transform himself. This can be difficult when the mind is constantly distracted by sights and sounds that arrest and cater to the senses. Living in a society filled with manmade creations can harden the heart by removing us from nature.

The increasing dependency upon technology can as easily weaken the will and crush the imagination as it sparks inventiveness and motivates. Science fiction is filled with modern morality plays encouraging man to grow by making good use of his inventions while warning if he does not they will overtake his life because of his sloth.

Simply put, in terms of physical health technology has so changed life in the United States that health clubs and gymnasiums are large businesses. The manual labor of everyday living used to give the body the exercise it needs to maintain good health. Widespread technology has changed that. From washing machines that replaced scrub boards and rocks to food preservatives and grocery stores that replaced family gardens and canning, modern conveniences have changed the kind and therefore the quality of life we live.

The greatest change technology has brought is not comfort, security, or even global communication. The greatest change is in man's relationship with time. How technology has altered our concept of time is either our glory or our ruin. Technology can seem to give us more time when in reality it does not. What it does give us is freedom. The full day we would have spent washing now requires an hour. The constant vigilance of planting, weeding, tending, harvesting, preserving food is no longer required in order to survive.

Change is inevitable. It is the nature of the physical world. The more we understand change, the more we embrace it, and the more we cause it in ourselves the healthier we become. From understanding comes the control man has always desired.

Technology has freed our time by fulfilling survival needs. What we do in those free hours, how we use them determines the degree of benefit received. We can become "couch potatoes" in consciousness and physical stature or we can enrich our lives by volunteering that time to teach a child to read, collect household items for those who are needy, or minister to the sick. The choices are apparent. The first is reactive, degenerative to mind and body, and in that harmful to the soul. The latter is responsive, stimulating to mind and body and fulfilling to the soul. Inadvertently technology is offering the opportunity to advance spiritual evolution if only we will respond. When we change ourselves first we have the wisdom and vision to work wonders in the world.

The power is in resurrecting our own consciousness.

Resurrecting consciousness may be simpler than you imagine.

Ideas of self-development, self-awareness, self-control are becoming more common. Every magazine has at least one article that expresses the virtues of a positive mental attitude.

Consider, for instance, this headline in a popular Sunday newspaper-magazine: *"Want to live longer, better, and wiser?"* (March 20, 1994 *Parade Magazine*) In answer to this question the article went on to list ten pointers:

1 Cherish your choices and maintain control of your own life.

2 Commit yourself to your passions in work and love—and embrace the conflicts and juggling involved.

3 Do more than one thing well.

4 Stop being afraid of real intimacy,

5 Risk being yourself, who you really are.

6 Pay attention to what's going on, the changes in your body and the outside world, the feelings of those you love and those with whom you work.

7 Risk new things, risk new ways, risk failing, risk mistakes, risk pain.

8 Use technologies and medical advances if they enhance or sustain your life—but beware of those that take choice away from you.

9 Be a part of the changing community.

10 Live it all.

Always vigilant for Universal Truth, I searched for what these pointers shared. What did all ten have in common? The answer was timeless and direct: all require us to change.

I have long admired the visionary work of Elizabeth Kubler-Ross. Dr. Kubler-Ross has devoted her life to understanding the most mysterious change man experiences – leaving physical existence; dying. How her research fit into what I was researching in intuitive realities was quite phenomenal.

By assisting, aiding, and counseling dying patients, Dr. Kubler-Ross insightfully identified five stages that are universally significant. When I was first presented with this years ago, I could see these stages of awareness experienced by those who are facing death also arise throughout our lives *anytime we are fighting change.*

Think about it. What happens when something unexpected occurs in our lives? All of a sudden someone whom we depended upon is no longer there. That is a physical change. Or we discover our company is moving its operations to another city and if we are going to stay with that company we have to move too. That's a change. Or a new baby arrives in our household restructuring our lives, that's a change. We tend to fight these kinds of normal experiences. Even when change is eagerly anticipated, the reality is often difficult because we don't know how to internalize the change. We have yet to learn to resurrect our own consciousness.

The fact that our choices in life bring us a succession of experiences where we can grow and mature in our understanding of change is one of the great reasons for our spirits to live in this physical world.

Dr. Kubler-Ross learned why death is so painful for most people. First they deny. Rather than embrace the spiritual life ahead of them, these people desperately clung to physical life, even through escalating debilitation. Then comes the anger, the bargaining, and the depression. Even in the ruin of life as they knew it, patients would cling to what is familiar rather than openly embrace the inevitable release that comes. They fight change, in stages, making the death process very, very difficult for them. Eventually that embrace, acceptance as Dr. Kubler-Ross calls it, does arrive and often people wonder what took them so long.

When accepting mortality takes a long time, it comes from how you have lived, how you have constructed your thinking during your life. If you've made it your habit to make life hard then that pattern will rule when it comes time for you to end physical life. For instance if you're the kind of person whose first reaction to a suggestion is "well, I don't know" or "I doubt it" or "I don't do that" then you practice denial. The "not me" consciousness. It's like someone who is aware of eating too much but keeps on feasting as if a famine that never arrives is coming. His denial will lead to physical health problems associated with the reason for his denial. Or someone in their youth who believes they can abuse their body with drugs and not "get caught" by liver disease or cancer. "Not me."

The need to change is omnipresent. It is everywhere around us and within us. To fight change is like a skier halfway down a mountain who disregarded the warnings of avalanche whose denial gives way to torrents of anger and pitiful bargains directed toward a God he does not know. Denial, anger, bargaining, and depression are what make change unbearable. They are attitudes we all possess, ways of thinking that keep us from facing the challenges in our life. But only temporarily.

Metaphysically speaking, the postponement of acceptance is in direct proportion to the degree of attachment to the physical world we have practiced during the life. Simply stated, the person who possesses a devout spiritual faith has lived his life believing in divine and supernatural realities. Such a person does not postpone thinking about his physical mortality. It is integrated into his concept of life and death which is one part of a much greater existence. The body is a shell that temporarily encases the soul. When it is shed, the soul or spirit will be freed. Physical death is a time for rejoicing for those invested in religious principles. And any change which brings us closer to spiritual consciousness is to be highly prized.

Looking forward to change may seem alien. But let's put it in the context of an everyday experience, perhaps one you have experienced – wisdom teeth. I heard the tales from "You'll start displaying wisdom when those teeth come in" to "Your life's half over when your wisdom teeth come in." In my twenties I began to experience pain in my jaw. Often the gums in the back of my mouth were inflamed and tender. There was no decay so I surmised my wisdom teeth were making themselves known.

As the weeks went by irritation turned into pain. It was difficult to eat. Sometimes my other teeth hurt and I could visually see only a small corner of two teeth, the remainder was hidden in the skin that stretches to form the back portion of your mouth. In other words it just didn't look like there was enough room for those teeth to fit. After a year of discomfort, a year of denial, I finally admitted I needed help. This admittance was a point of acceptance that initiated action and over several months I had three of the wisdom teeth pulled. That left one upper tooth that wasn't bothering me and showed no movement until a couple years later.

When it started to move, I was painfully aware of its presence. Having been through the pulling of the other three it seemed inevitable to me what would eventually occur. However my life at the time was not conducive to stopping to tend to body malfunctions. I was constantly on the road, three hundred and sixty-five days a year and I was attached to having "my" dentist do the work. So I fought the change.

I'd been through the experience three times before so I knew what was ahead. Although it pulling teeth is not a pleasant experience it is tolerable. I was not facing an unknown situation. What I faced, with the removal of this last wisdom tooth, was a change in consciousness that would affect the rest of my life. Since the earlier extractions, I had made many changes in attitude and lifestyle. I had learned a great deal about the connection between mind and body, including Dr. Kubler-Ross's work. For me this simple passage in life became the stimulus for Self revelation for I clearly saw why I fought change and more importantly what I could do to stop fighting and start making change happen.

Within a matter of hours I moved from one stage to the next beginning with the first step of fighting change: denial. "It's not that bad." "Oh, well, maybe I'll wake up tomorrow and it will stop bothering me." "Maybe it will just stop where it is. After all it hasn't moved for years. And if it stops it won't cause any more problems." I realized that the tooth was indeed there and it was moving. It was pressing on the tooth next to it, causing it to hurt. Even if there was room for that wisdom tooth in my mouth, there was nothing present on the bottom to stop its movement because the bottom tooth had been removed years earlier. A good way to recognize areas of denial in your thinking is to hear the "NO's!" that come out of your own mouth – not me, not now, do not, should not, and so on. Ignorance, persistent and stubborn ignoring of what is happening, is the consciousness of someone who denies change. Change, however, does not go away, it makes its needs known. Pain is the result of ignorance.

Bothering escalated into hurt and my efforts to ignore were useless. Yes, I could take an aspirin to interfere with messages of pain being sent to my brain, but such action was in direct opposition to my beliefs and practices. I knew what I needed to do, but first I got mad. "I don't have time for this!" First I was mad at the tooth, then I was mad at myself. "I should have had it done earlier." I had gone through this three times already and

I knew it really wasn't all that bad when you really get down do it. But ... "if I'd already done it then I wouldn't have to be thinking about it and taking time to do it now." Blame is a characteristic of anger, the second step in fighting change. I threw the blame on myself, many times people cast it on others which prolongs the battle often hurting others in the process. As with all blame, it solves nothing and wounds everything because it is a poor-spirited version of responsibility. I had learned a great deal about responsibility as freedom so I didn't stay in anger.

Fairly quickly I moved into bargaining. "Okay, I'll go to the dentist – the next time I'm in town. Maybe in the meantime if I massage my gums it will push on through and be okay. Maybe if I start saying what's on my mind instead of holding back it will help. Maybe if I take vitamins the pain will go away." I came up with all kind of creative thoughts. In retrospect, I marveled at the waste of time and creative energy that could have spent in endeavors beneficial to others and much more fulfilling for myself. That's the quality of bargaining though. It does move you forward because you are considering alternatives, but the progress is in large part only intellectual. Somewhere, sometime, you will need to commit to action and test your hypothesis. Bargaining is easy to identify in your thinking because it is characterized by "if......then" lines of thinking. During all my creative fervor the wisdom tooth was still there, still causing me pain, and it was not going to go away unless I caused it to.

That realization led to the fourth stage in the fight which is depression. Although before my studies in applied metaphysics depression was a common demon I battled, this depression didn't last long. In fact, by now I was finding myself entertained because I was learning so much about me. I was going through these stages with awareness, identifying each one as they appeared. The accompanying revelations were awesome. Depression sounded like "Why couldn't I be like my mother?" Sounds strange? It won't when you hear that my mother never had wisdom teeth. I was depressed that I didn't inherit her lack of wisdom teeth, because if I had I wouldn't be going through all of this. Sounds funny, doesn't it? It did to me too and by placing self-pity in a more proper perspective I was free of its considerable tentacles. Depression is characterized by the open-ended question "why?" When you can place why in perspective you are free to pursue an answer or invent one of your own. You are free to face the reality of your life and learn the lesson before you.

People go through these stages every day. At any given time they can dig their heels in, stubbornly refusing to move. So society has a bigot, someone who has been stuck in denial for years. Or a bully, someone who has remained in anger for years. Or a con artist, someone whose sole approach to life is bargaining. Or a victim, someone who has been depressed for years. These people are dying. Maybe not in the sense that they are on their deathbeds, their bodies riddled by disease but I will guarantee you the seeds for that demise are already sown in the painful attitudes they abide. While they tarry, indulging human frailty and weakness, their soul is suffering. Their innate urge to spiritually grow is dying. It is dying to be expressed. It wants health and it wants wholeness. The conscious mind says no! no! And we wonder why we become ill.

The soul desires resurrection. Our outer selves, the waking physical mind, must align its desire with those that provide it a spark of life. The conscious mind must readily accept change with hope and expectation.

There is a certain resolve that comes at the end of conflict. Giving up the fight opens the door to seeking accord. Acceptance, as Dr. Kubler-Ross' dying patients found and as I discovered with my wisdom tooth, is the key to that door. In both cases what was being accepted is the fact that a physical change was in order. For the person at the end of physical life, acceptance is surrendering into death's embrace freeing the soul, something we will speak more of later. For the person moving through life, acceptance is forfeiting self-imposed limitations thus freeing the creative mind to learn, grow, and evolve.

I decided to stop playing games with myself and do what needed to be done.

The most enlightening part of this experience came not with getting to the point of physical action and resolve, it came with the transformation in consciousness I was making. Spiritual growth, mental excellence, and physical health have always been important to me. They are real needs in my life. Being able to see how I sabotaged myself in these areas was exciting because I now had the upper hand. I was no longer dependent upon circumstances to dictate my need for change. I learned self-knowledge enables me to exert self-control when and where I need it.

I now recognized my real need is for internal change, the kind of elevation of awareness that resurrects consciousness. What I was learning about consciousness and the skills in reasoning and intuition I was building

– applied metaphysics – would be put to the test in a new way. For by releasing myself from the self-defeating, closed-minded thinking associated with the stages of fighting change, I was presented with a simple question, "What change do you want to make?" Change had ceased to be an enemy to defend myself from, and had become something to create that would bring fulfillment to my life.

What came next are the five steps to making a change, indeed creating transformation, in yourself and your life. I call them the "five stages of living life."

Awareness was my reward when I stopped giving myself trouble by fighting change. I could with ease admit the change that needed to take place. I hadn't been able to relieve my body of discomfort. It was physically painful and mentally distracting. I needed help. I admitted, "I can't do this alone." With this statement came the awareness that I needed the counsel of someone who has made oral hygiene their life's specialty, a professional. I needed a dentist's service to make the change that would restore my body to health. I was no longer afraid of admitting "Change has to occur in order for my body to be healthy." Awareness of the change that needs to take place is the first step of living life.

I knew from my studies that change would free the considerable mental energy I consumed fighting pain to be used in more beneficial endeavors. Being free from pain, both mental and physical, would give me a fresh outlook and renewed motivation to live life well. I was beginning to form a desire for the impending change. Desire, the mind's capacity to reach for what it lacks, to draw what it needs, is the second stage of consciousness that creates change. I wanted to think clearly again. I no longer wanted to endure a condition that I believed could be readily remedied.

Belief in a productive and positive outcome creates a well formed desire, an image that includes the intention of its maker in the ideal to be attained. This is what creates a seed idea. It is the combining of desire and will. The catalyst for the two to merge can be described as decision, the third stage. In the saga of my wisdom tooth it sounded like this, "Okay, no more excuses, no more procrastination, the next time I'm in Springfield I'll make the dental appointment and I'll do it." Decision. A commitment to action that will produce the change desired.

Now came one of the busiest stages, creating a plan. Setting an available time and day then calling the dentist to schedule an appointment was only the beginning of my planning. I wanted to be mentally and emotionally prepared as well. For this I drew on past experience, my own and others. I remembered a story a friend of mine told me about her dental experience. She went to the dentist to have a tooth removed several days before a scheduled speaking engagement. The doctor worked on that tooth and worked on that tooth, for ten minutes, trying to get it out. Finally she said she realized what she was doing. She was holding on to the tooth, mentally holding on to it. She did not want to lose it.

She put up her hand and said, "Stop." The dentist really did not know what to do because he had no idea what *she* was doing. What she was doing was a type of mental accounting, reviewing her attitudes. She knew she was refusing to let go of the tooth so she took a couple of minutes to relax , changing her consciousness. She came to terms with her attachment, deciding it was okay, it was time to let it go. She told the doctor she was ready. He went in and the tooth came right out. He couldn't understand it. It baffled him. Always respect the power of your mind. And use what you know. That was the lesson here.

By this time, I knew that thought is cause. I knew it is my attitude in life, not circumstances, that determines my pleasure or sorrow. My perspective of life is the source of my own optimism and enthusiasm or my pessimism and apathy. I knew my attitude immediately affects my body, learning how to cure years of recurring headaches and menstrual cramps had proved that. I was aware that my attitude played a major role in previous dental visits. Wanting this experience to be as painless as possible, I employed mental imagery so it would be very easy for this tooth to be released. Part of my plan was letting go of this tooth so it would come out real easily.

Imagination played as important a part in my planning as memory. My future – beyond the physical change of losing a tooth – also became part of my plan. As far as I could mentally see, I imaged what I wanted. Healing was a big part of my plan. I *prepared* to heal. I knew this change would be abrupt, placing undue stress upon the body. I knew the body would heal naturally according to Universal Law. This process would require time. I wanted to cooperate with the healing and I wanted to accelerate it. I had many things to do in my life. I wanted to speed my recovery and in order for that to occur I had to prepare for it. That's what I did, mentally, emotionally, and physically. One of my physical preparations, which you might find useful at some time, was drinking pineapple juice. I had learned from countless Intuitive Health Analyses that pineapple juice causes a proper acid-alkaline balance in the mouth that is conducive to healing.

When I did finally take action, the change was relatively painless and very quick in recovery and healing. The entire process went exactly as I'd imaged it. In fact hours later, following a two hour drive and long after the effects of Novacaine had dissipated, I was teaching a class. I have used an example from my own learning to paint a picture of how we fight change and, I trust, I have imparted how truly easy it is to make changes, to cause health and wholeness in every area of our lives.

Resurrecting my consciousness made all the difference for me in this situation and countless life situations since then. In every creative endeavor, be it writing a book, giving birth to a child, drawing plans for a campus chapel, or initiating a global effort like the Universal Hour of Peace, I have employed these five stages of living life fully: awareness, desire, decision, plan, and action. I have taught others to use them as well, with amazing results. These stages resurrect your consciousness beyond what may be holding you back, restricting and limiting your creative power. As we use the mind's innate visualizing power—putting the mind into directive action, on purpose and with purpose—we find the conditions in our physical lives are easy to embrace and transform.

Intuitive Health Analysis can quicken the process. Each analysis identifies what needs to change for there to be restoration, rejuvenation, balance, and wholeness in the system. As you have learned, suggestions for those changes are also given. Typically, people immediately respond to some part of the analysis, usually an answer to a question in an area of concern. Like the woman who wanted to know if there was any physical reason for her not bearing a child or the man who wanted to know if he had Lyme's disease or the parent who asked about his child's persistent bedwetting. The reason people seek an Intuitive Health Analysis is the area in their consciousness where they are most open to change, and so they are the most attentive and responsive to what is related concerning that area. The rest of the report is too often left alone. It does not receive equal scrutiny and so what it has to offer is only potential. Too many times I hear people say, "You know the health analysis you did for me two, three, or five years ago said something about this condition but I didn't pay any attention to it at the time."

I know how much someone can gain from an Intuitive Health Analysis. It can be the difference between restoration and resurrection, and compromise and settling. For years, as a teacher and psi counselor, I have been able to aid people to see what they might have overlooked, to create actions that cause progressive change to wellness. Recently at our world headquarters we began offering a forum that teaches how to fully utilize intuitively-accessed information. Spiritual Initiation Sessions are designed to teach people how to embrace and cause change in themselves, encouraging them to go directly to acceptance then move through the stages that will resurrect their consciousness.

Genuine health is only possible in the context of healthy relationships, healthy communities, and a nurturing connection with nature. Mainstream advocates have come to realize and accept this timeless Truth. During Spiritual Initiation Sessions, hosted on the campus of the College of Metaphysics in Missouri, you experience all three.

Spiritual Initiation Sessions seek to introduce you to new ways of thinking, living, and being. These weekends elevate your spirit, enrich your mind, warm your heart, and nourish your body by creating the atmosphere of Spiritual, Intuitive Man. In the course of forty-eight hours, you eat, sleep, talk, meditate, laugh, and sometimes even cry with people you met on Friday evening. What you discover is the commonality of our hopes and dreams. These go beyond any physical differences that people might turn into barriers. What we have in common opens us to addressing each other as souls. You attend a Spiritual Initiation Session not with strangers but with spiritual friends with whom you have much in common.

Under the guidance of a mentor, sessions teach you to apply spiritual principles in your thinking, choices, and actions. Of the seven topics offered throughout the year, two are centered around Intuitive Health Analyses: *First Opinion*, on a personal analysis, and *First Teacher*, on a child's analysis. The insights gained from the inner levels of consciousness are explored and developed under the guidance of a mentor who holds a Doctorate of Metaphysics and who has taught hundreds of people for two decades or more. Dr. Pam Blosser, who serves as analysis coordinator at SOM World Headquarters, has mentored these sessions since their inception. With almost two decades of experience with the analyses, she has helped thousands schedule, receive, and utilize the insights gained through intuitively accessed information.

"The Intuitive Health Analysis is a place for people to identify where they have lost their power," Dr. Blosser says. "They have given their power over to something else and this is what the analysis describes. It's not a personal judgment on them, although upon first hearing an analysis people sometimes hear only what is going wrong, after all this is what is requested in these analyses – *'relate all disorders as seen....'*. Following the description of the problem, each analysis includes suggestions in all systems for correction and healing.

"It's important to go beyond initial reactions because the analysis offers people very real ways to become whole and healthy. It can help them to identify where they lost power and where they lost really — I want to say spirit. They kind of like died at that point. The suggestions in the analysis are there to bring the power back to them and help them to renew their spirit. When people receive the information with an attitude of 'where have I lost the power, where have I lost my spirit,' then it's a much more compassionate way of looking at themselves. Then I think they can be more open to hearing everything the analysis has to say without feeling like it's criticism. The way the *First Opinion* and *First Teacher* sessions are designed gives people every opportunity to comprehend and utilize the full value of the Intuitive Health Analysis."

The weekends are two days of focused self-exploration. They are a spiritual journey that begins on Friday evening and culminates at a supernatural destination on Sunday afternoon. Some participants experience miraculous healing; all receive the information and instruction that places them on a path that will cause healing in themselves and in their relations with others. People are transformed because they have spent hours deeply contemplating the meaning of their analysis while implementing the changes suggested in their dealings with others and their daily activities. By Sunday, they are well on their way to causing a *permanent* healing in themselves.

How this all comes about draws upon both the five stages of death and the five stages of living life. In a weekend you learn how to apply these principles in your own life for healing.

You do indeed learn how to resurrect your consciousness.

A Spiritual Journey toward Resurrection

People come from all over the world to the small hamlet in the beautiful countryside in the heart of the United States. They are on a quest. A quest for answers. A quest for enrichment of soul and body. A quest for peace.

And their quest is fulfilled.

Each *First Opinion* weekend is a spiritual journey. The focus is wholeness. The journey begins by imaging being the healthiest you can be. Guided imagery, meditation, and discussion this first evening is devoted to you at your best, your optimum, your zenith. It prepares you for the intuitive information you will receive in your analysis following yoga, meditation, and breakfast tomorrow morning.

You witness your analysis being given and are invited to ask questions. Following enlightening conversation with the intuitive reporter and conductor, your mentor aids you in resurrecting your consciousness to wholeness. This process is known as a psi awakening. Your mentor directs you to choose one outstanding suggestion from your analysis, one phrase that has special meaning for you, for you will use this as a focal point throughout the weekend. Noting what you are changing *from* accelerates this process. In every analysis there is at least one phrase that serves to mentally arouse you each time you fall back into the unproductive pattern of thinking, the old habit. Like a mental alarm clock, it awakens you to the need for change. Knowing how to transform your consciousness completes the psi awakening.

During the Spiritual Initiation Session each person is present when the analyses are conducted so they are in a position to support each others' changes, offer encouragement or ideas that are compatible to the new ways of thinking. In one session, "feeling burdened" is one woman's mental alarm. Thoughts like, "It's hard, it's really hard to do. I can't handle any more." For another, it is when she is inattentive, when she doesn't know what her mind is doing. Thoughts like, "Did I miss something? What did you say? Where's that turn I'm supposed to make?" The need is to learn how to identify her thoughts, still her mind and identify her thoughts. This is her psi awakening. Another one's alarm is when she resists doing something she knows is in her best interest. Like exercising and she is saying "I don't really want to do that." Another's awakening is the positive action of sharing. His habit was stopping himself from talking because he was thinking he would hurt someone's feelings or it would bother somebody. His mental alarm is disturbed silence; his awakening, saying something when he would otherwise refuse, to give rather than pull away. The choices of mental alarms are very specific so the psi awakening can begin immediately and build throughout the weekend with the help of all participants. The interaction becomes rich – people helping people – and the results are astounding for everyone present. By the time the weekend is over, new modes of responding, healthy ways of thinking, are already established as participants return to their homes.

One participant, a college student, described this synergy well, "We all listed the productive suggestions the health analysis gave and we were going to focus on a productive suggestion the remainder of the weekend. One of the women was having a hard time defining her focus so we were trying to help her. We all had a bit of a hard time finding a suggestion that she could apply and know she was applying.

"I had taken some really good notes on everybody's health analysis and this came in handy because even though her analysis didn't say 'give her a suggestion for building her will' it said 'this one has a weak will and tends to let others make decisions for her.' So I suggested she make choices all weekend and build her will. And she did – what food she was going to eat first, was she going to eat it slowly or quickly, or give it attention or talk. It was a learning experience for all of us. Neither she nor the rest of us had thought, realized, the continuous series of choices that creates the kind of day we have.

"I gave that suggestion even though my initial fearful thought was 'that's silly, the analysis didn't say it.' Looking back now, I can see I was using the information in my own health report - *'to cease allowing fear to rule my thoughts by valuing my thoughts and courageously expressing them without attachment'* – to aid her. This reciprocal benefit happened quite a bit, where people would use their own analysis to make an internal change while aiding other people to use theirs."

This willingness to help others accentuates the depth of the session. It also encourages openness, honesty, trust, and thus self-revelation. Those who are prepared to give from the very beginning are the ones who receive throughout the weekend. In one session such a person set the tone for the entire session. During introductions the first night when asked if she had any children she kind of hesitated and then she said, "Yes I have one daughter who is 29." She went on to say she knows when people ask her if she has any children there is this discomfort, and she wanted to go beyond it. She said when she was 16 years old she had a daughter who she gave up because she didn't want to marry the father. She knew it would be disastrous and she thought that was the best thing for the child. Soon after that she met her current husband. They have a good life and just a couple of years ago she came in contact with her daughter who is a wonderful person. It has turned out really well where her daughter really loves her and her husband. This was a lot to tell somebody, particularly people you have not previously known but this is the caliber of these sessions. The closeness, the trust, the desire to heal and be healed is a very powerful force during these sessions.

There is always a strong group consciousness present. Everybody is motivated from desire to cause a change. The attitude is "I really want to take this now and use it and apply it to my life." This produces an enormous amount of energy directed toward ideals that are becoming more defined moment by moment. This raises everybody's level of desire. It supports everybody's commitment to do, to use, to gain. The psychic energy is phenomenally powerful.

Those who are initially more retiring or shy often make the most dramatic transformations during the weekend. One college professor reached a point where he "decided to surrender his ego. To open up and to learn." It was magical because it stimulated everyone else present to take a similar step. During one of the enactments, purposeful interaction settings, he decided he was going to talk freely because he realized he'd been really quiet and withdrawn. Before this transition, when others would try to converse with him he would pull further and further in. But after surrendering his ego, participants reported that he opened more and more and more and more until he was "just very comfortable by the end of the weekend," "very easy to tell people what his thoughts and feelings were." This was a miraculous healing for this man. And a spontaneous healing for the group.

Each session member deepens the experience of each other member. What is personally received can alter dreams and ambitions, perceptions and prejudices. The freedom experienced as truth is realized is the thrill of the journey and the stimulus to continue. Consider the following participants' experiences as seen through the eyes of the session's mentor.

The Engineer

In the course of her analysis the Engineer asked, *"How can this one change the thinking to embrace consistently, surpassing previously accomplished ideals? This one says I feel like I am not equipped to top or go beyond some of the ideals I have created."* The answer that the intuitive reporter gave was *"This is not true. This would be the first step is to recognize this is a lie in this one's thinking. This one is equipped to accomplish anything she can imagine, otherwise she would not be capable of imagining it."*

She said when she heard this it was such a relief that what she was telling herself was not true. Those ideas of not being good enough, or being ill prepared, or not wanted were lies. This cleansed years of self-doubt.

Close to the time of closing the session, the mentor asked participants, "How are you different?" The Engineer said she was relieved. The word she used, or the phrase, was "embracing her own love." The analysis suggested she *"immerse the self in the love that this one experiences"* in order to become aware of the limitlessness of her capabilities. This was quite a transformation because at first this concept was difficult for the Engineer so the mentor created a situation whereby the Engineer could indeed immerse herself in the kind of love that she gives others and see its immediate effects.

Remember the Engineer wanted to know how she could change her thinking to surpass what she had done before. The mentor had the Engineer choose an ideal she wanted to accomplish. The Engineer, who often teaches continuing education courses, chose a class she was considering offering. When considering this ideal, she was filled with doubts that she would have enough people registered to warrant the school continuing to offer her course. When she was asked to add to this goal the new idea about immersing herself in love, she had a difficult time. She was talking real slowly and softly. So all the session participants sat down. Everyone was drawn to her from their own desire to help her, assist her in accomplishing her ideal rather than her fears.

In a flash of inspiration that only arises from the synergy of these sessions, the mentor envisioned an experience that would help the Engineer to realize the power of her thoughts. The mentor instructed the participants, "Okay, we are people out here and we are just walking around, and we are people who might be in your class. If [the Engineer] says something that is attractive to you then you can walk closer to her. If she says something that isn't attractive to you then you walk farther away." The Engineer started talking. It was funny at first because she was saying "I'm really a good teacher" so everybody started coming toward her, "but I don't know if I can handle that many people" and the people would turn around, walking away. This was an obvious illustration of the Universal Law of Attraction, the concept behind "birds of a feather flock together" and "like attracts like." Most participants could readily grasp this, but the Engineer was still holding onto her limitations. She had yet to cause a transition in her thinking. As her analysis pointed out, *"...this one will need to cause there to be motivation and discipline within this one's thinking and life. We see that as this one will begin to embrace the soul's urge for growth, this one will find a freedom that she has long sought and at times abandoned."*

As she continued describing her doubts people just wandered about because she wasn't saying anything that was really attractive, she wasn't disciplining her mind to remain upon what she had to give that was valuable to others. She was doing what the analysis had described, *"We see that there is a very strong urge within this one to be different than other people, to be outstanding in different fields, to give something that others cannot. And we see that by refusing to admit the ways in which this one is unique and the understandings that she holds, and the talents that this one possesses, this one does deny the Self the capability of manifesting this difference."* She still wasn't realizing how the change in how she uses her imagination is the attractive force that will ensure her success. So the mentor had everyone sit down. Everyone offered her encouragement by describing the qualities she displayed which were attractive. She improved slightly, becoming a bit more positive and alive in expressing her ideas.

The mentor knew that the Engineer was still missing the essence of the health analysis's suggestion so she asked everyone present, "Whether you've known [the Engineer] for a long time or have known her for a short time, you've all experienced her love. Is that right?" Everybody agreed. So the mentor had the Engineer stand and had all the participants surround her. Then the mentor said, "Now give her the love back that you have experienced receiving from her." Everyone stepped forward and touched her. She was in the middle of all these people hugging her.

That created a memory that will last her lifetime.

The Computer Technician

The computer technician's analysis began *"We see a kind of insecurity within this one that arises from lack of experience. We see that this one tends to intellectualize or to grasp concepts very quickly with the thinking. We see that this one has a great capacity for memory and attention, and yet we see that this one has yet to coordinate these with the imagination in order to produce reasoning."* He demonstrated this from the moment of his arrival. His intellectualizing, rationalizing, was quite practiced. For instance he would say things like, "I've thought that my fear thoughts were real thoughts and that in fact they are just fear thoughts. I need to see them for what they are." His repetitive use of words might at first sound deeply thoughtful but upon closer examination they begin and end at the same point without traveling anywhere. Thus the words reflect a repetitive train of thought, memorized, which leaves him where he is rather than moving him forward in life.

His insecurity was revealed time and again in what he had to say. His words conveyed the idea that he thinks he should know something already because he has information about it in his brain. He lacks the confidence that comes with knowing something because he has yet to use the information in experience. This is a common problem in this technological age where the immediate transference of global knowledge, the information superhighway, is held in higher regard than individual wisdom. As Albert Einstein remarked, "Imagination is more important than knowledge." The Computer Tech's analysis said, *"The true difficulty that this one experiences is the need to put the ideas that this one holds to the test in order to cause there to be understandings, and eventually wisdom."* This was the key that would help the Computer Tech transform his life for the root of his problems with others lay in his tendency to misuse his imagination to *"build false ideas of this one's ineffectiveness, or difficulty with people, or incompetence, a string of imagined negative qualities that actually do not even exist."* Putting himself on the line everywhere in his life became a theme to bring his imagination under his control.

The beginning of this occurred when early in the weekend the Tech said he just needed to quit thinking so much. During his analysis he had asked, *"Why do I sometimes feel very tired and how can I have more energy?"* The answer: *"This one thinks too much and it is very wearing upon the self, mentally, emotionally, and physically."* Throughout the weekend, whenever this wearing became apparent, the participants would say, "you are thinking too much." "Stop thinking so much." This gave him a point of security because he began to realize he doesn't have to make judgments about himself. He doesn't have to live out his fears. He can recognize that he now has information that he can *"put to the test."*

The mentor's suggestion was as soon as he receives a new piece of information to imagine immediately how he can apply that somewhere in his life. After the weekend he remarked, "One of the things that my analysis suggested was to combine imagination with my attention and memory to form reasoning. All weekend long, I was practicing different ways to use reasoning, to imagine different things. Especially the big part that my health analysis focused on was that I created all these little fears. It's like they're little fears that I immediately, just because I thought them, think that they're already real. And so it's like I might have a fear that someone's going to react to me in a certain way because they did before. And so it stops me from saying something to them or doing something that I want to do to fulfill a desire. During the weekend I was realizing where maybe I was afraid to talk about something or afraid to give something to somebody and I'd be like 'No! I'm going to change this.' And I would imagine a different way of being."

Having an immediate response gave him a sense of relief and a kind of empowerment. Those are the words he used at the end of the weekend. Relief and he felt empowered. He had the power now. The power was back in his hands.

The Broker's Assistant

"This one has created a very strong persona...this has become this one's focal point and this one's security, and therefore it is difficult for this one to be able to imagine being able to explore different parts of the Self; being able to as this one sees it, reveal different parts of her Self" her report began. An interesting correlation arose for the assistant because the Health Analysis she received during the session was her second one in a month. The earlier analysis described her difficulty as "being dishonest". The session analysis was a continuation of the same theme, the "persona" was the point of dishonesty.

She described a situation between her and her mother when she was five years old. She wanted to wear a pink silk shirt and her mother didn't want her to wear it because the assistant had outgrown the shirt. From a five-year-old's perspective she didn't understand that. She just wanted to wear this shirt because she liked it. Ever since then she has held on to this. As her analysis said, *"We see that this one values the emotions more than the thinking; therefore this one tends to judge with the emotions which causes this one's perceptions to many times be in error."*

Now, fifteen years later, she is on her own. When she and her mother go shopping, anything that her mother seems to like or wants her to try on, even if she too likes it, the assistant will just say no. She's defiant. She is not reasoning, she reacts. This became apparent when the assistant said that she secretly liked some of her mother's choices and were she by herself she might even get them. But because her mother suggested it, she just absolutely says "No, I don't like that." *"As has been stated, this one does approach life from an emotional basis. This one tends to react to the environment and to make her judgements based on what she feels, rather than to think, to reason, to look for facts, form beliefs, and transcend these beliefs into knowing."* She thinks her mother is trying to control her and think of her as a little girl and she doesn't want to be a little girl anymore. One of the other participants suggested that if she really wanted a change then she would need to begin acting like an adult. It was a shining example of how the assistant has *"has a very strong emotional base, and that this one does project this to others."*

By virtue of the fact that the first problem cited in the analysis was something about the persona, it made sense the assistant would find the greatest challenge or difficulty in the weekend. In receiving the analysis, seeing the concepts, and responding to them, changes would occur "to" her persona. By the end of the session she said I am more aware, she at least has some awareness of what she is doing. She may not be able to identify when she is doing it yet, but she does know this is what she does. She knew she hadn't made a dramatic change but she had the beginning of making some changes. The secret she has yet to learn is she doesn't have to change the persona. She doesn't have to lose it and that's her greatest fear. What she must do is add to it. As she adds to it, she'll discover she gains freedom by adding to and being different, expressing different parts of herself. By experiencing more, becoming deeper and more multifaceted, the defiant or limiting parts of her persona, she'll see differently and even be able to let go of them as she matures.

The Building Contractor

He said when he was five years old he saw his brother floating on the ceiling. His brother was in Viet Nam and within a week they got a telegram saying that he had died. Well, being five years old he thought he had caused his brother to die.

Then as he was growing up his mother was prone to declaring she would not die until all her sons were married. She said it over and over again. The Building Contractor was the youngest son, and the last one to marry. Before his wedding, he had a premonition that his mother was going to die. The lady he married had the same vision. They didn't tell each other until after his mother died, during his wedding reception. This time he realized he hadn't caused his mother to die. He knew that if he had said anything to his family ahead of time, or even said it afterwards, they would have said, "Well, why didn't you do something about it." He knew that his mother needed to go and she was waiting for him to get married and that was it. But he knew that if he said this to his family they wouldn't have understood it.

Then there's his aunt. His aunt was his father's favorite sister. She was dying and his father was in Canada. They called his father. She was waiting until he got there to die. The same idea. After he got there she was conscious enough where they talked to each other and then she became unconscious. The father had to make the choice of whether to leave her on a life support system or let her go. The family was divided, some people said yes and some people said no. The Building Contractor didn't say anything. Although he wanted to say no, he said nothing.

As he revealed the tragedies in his life, it was easy to see how the analysis had pinpointed the common cause within him: *"We see completion to be very difficult for this one. We see this manifests in every area of this one's life. We see that this one has difficulty in bringing associations, projects, conversations to a point of culmination. We see there is a pain associated with parting. There is a sorrow that underlies this one's thinking and emotions in regards to ending something and this is why this one tends to avoid at all cost completing anything. As a result this one leaves many loose ends in the life."*

Following a guided imagery he talked about how his dad and his family had treated his aunt dying. He was asked about how he completes things and he would not talk about how he completes things. He would only go on and on about his dad. So the mentor asked, "Now if your dad were to die tomorrow, would you have said everything you needed to say to him?" No, the Contractor answered.

The mentor asked, "Well if you were to die tomorrow would you have done everything you wanted to do?" No. That was his completion for that particular memory and train of thought. Life has gone on for his family, his dad, for him. He has unfinished business because completion is something he avoids at all costs. In his mind he sees that death is sometimes planned by the person. It's part of the process of life. But the kind of feedback he has gotten from other people has been "it's a terrible thing" and "it's so sorrowful" and "it's so traumatic." The whole idea of completing things he avoids. Regarding his emotions, his analysis said, *"We see that this one goes to extreme lengths to avoid closure, therefore this one believes that he spares himself and others unpleasantness or conflict or hurt. When in reality he is stealing from himself and others understanding, wisdom, and soul progression."* This was a shock to him. He had never considered the depths of how his reluctance to end conversations, associations, issues, affects others adversely.

Throughout the weekend the theme of death echoed in his discussion of life experiences. Slowly he began to recognize that every moment is a beginning and an ending unto itself. Every moment is the completion of one thing and the initiation of another. This was the beginning of seeing life differently. *"In order for this one to change the experience of life this one must be willing to transcend the unconscious pain that this one is trying to avoid and has spent the entire life avoiding. We see that this one must recognize the nature of life is change, the nature of existence is change, and therefore life is a continual series of hellos and goodbyes, beginning and endings, points of commencement and points of culmination."* He said he had changed through the weekend because he now could be committed. He felt more committed to completing the unfinished business from his past so he can live in the now.

The Bank Employee

We were curious upon first hearing the Bank Employee's analysis. *"We see immaturity in the mental system that arises because this one refuses to use the imagination in a productive fashion. We see that the ways that this one allows the imagination to wander is in a very scattered fashion and leaves very little for this one to build upon or to create with or to manifest. We see that this one has relied very heavily upon the environment for a source of discipline and structure and we see that this one has not adopted an attitude of learning so that this one could internalize a sense of structure and a sense of discipline in the Self. We see that this is very much needed to reach a state of mental and spiritual adulthood."* This made sense when we discovered that at 26 years of age the Bank Employee goes to her mother's house once a week to do her laundry.

Her analysis also indicated that she is ruled by her emotions. What she thinks and does is not only connected to her emotional reactions to the situations in her life but dictated by them. She recalled a time during physical adolescence when she and her friend were going to go cruising.

The friend's mother had told her daughter that she couldn't go cruising unless her room was cleaned. The friend defiantly didn't clean her room, so when it came time to go cruising her mother said, "No, you are not going to go cruising. You are going to clean up your room."

Angry, the friend went into her closet and started crying. The Bank Employee arrived to pick up her friend. She learns her friend is in her room. She goes upstairs, finds her friend in the closet and crawls in next to her. There they are, sitting in the closet, and the Bank Employee starts talking about her father which is a complete distraction from the intended goal of going cruising and not at all related to the friend cleaning her room. The friend starts talking about her own father and it becomes quite a sob story. *"We see that emotionally this one is given to tantrums. They are not always physically expressed, although they are at times, and we see that this is a reflection of the immaturity that has been spoken of. This one allows the emotions to carry the Self away and to leave this one without answers."* The Bank Employee gets sucked into her friend's emotional tantrum from the moment she arrives and only now years later does she realize she should have just said, "Look your mother said you need to clean your room before you go cruising. How come you didn't clean your room? I'm ready to go. But you're not ready. What's up?"

The fascinating reality for this woman is how she continues to allow her thinking to be scattered and her emotions muddied. During the weekend she had an opportunity to replay this memory with another participant. The woman playing her friend immediately responded to her role by sniffling and complaining, "Yeah, it's my father". Rather than act upon the hindsight she displayed moments before, the Bank Employee commiserates, "I can understand I have difficulties too." The friend says, "How do you have difficulties?" and the Bank Employee starts reliving her old perceptions of her dad. She is scattering her thoughts, getting even more sidetracked, and therefore emotionally involved. The mentor stopped her, asking, "Do you see what you just did?" Everybody laughed and she laughed saying, "I can't believe I just did it again."

Her analysis suggested stilling her mind so she can calm her emotions, *"In this way this one perpetuates a kind of emotional turmoil and confusion that this one will leave behind as she begins to strengthen her resolve and begins to gain understanding and wisdom. Would suggest that this one endeavor to take control of her emotions by learning to still the mind and from that, being able to calm them. A calm mind, a still mind does produce calmness mentally, emotionally and physically, therefore, would suggest that this one expand her consciousness to realize that it is not by going into the emotions and trying to wrestle with them and trying to make them do something that the control that is being spoken of will be gained. Rather it is by transcending the emotions and recognizing they are not a cause, they are an effect and working from a point of cause in how this one directs the thinking and life that this one has been living or move beyond it, or grow beyond it."*

Because the patterns are so well practiced, the Bank Employee has a difficult time identifying them as they arise unless someone around her is aware. With the flighty thinking and need for discipline, a physical means for detecting the need to direct attention was called for, *"It is important for this one to become aware of and develop a respect for the physical."* So her own body became her monitor, her alarm sounding the need for change. This was described in the analysis: *"...We see within the physical system that there is a kind of emotional quality to the body itself, therefore, the nervous system is highly reactive. We see that the body reacts very quickly to any kind of stimulus whether it is food, too much of some food or substance or too little of it whether it is sound or smell. We see that all the sensory nerves are raw, because this one allows the emotions to go wherever they want to go and does not direct the attention. The attention must be directed in order for the nervous system to work properly and be able to serve the body well as the means by which experience is collected. Therefore, the capacity for this one to be in the present moment and to direct the mind fully upon what is at hand is very important. This would aid in calming the body, the nerves and would aid greatly in the complete digestion of food which is often not digested at all. Therefore, the body is often malnourished..."* The analysis later suggested rolfing, a system of deep tissue massage therapies, could help her to gain self-awareness. This was encouraged, particularly by one who had experienced the therapy and could describe it to her. The mentor taught her several yoga postures that are helpful in focusing the mind's attention and she also gave instructions in relaxation and meditation to achieve a stilling of her consciousness. Of all the participants in this session, this woman had both the least amount of localized disorders and the greatest challenge in taking control of her own thinking and emotions.

The Public Defender

She was definitely ready to learn. She has a lot of physical difficulties. Her immune system is going. She has arthritis. Doctors are wanting to give her some kind of chemical that they use on cancer patients to help get rid of something that's in her joints that has to do with her arthritis. In part, this is how her Health Analysis described her condition and some of the suggestions she received: *"We see that there is a large degree of waste material that is held in the body that then becomes toxic to it. It wears upon the immune system, which is compromised at the present time period, and it does cause there to be at times aches and pains, or for instance times when lactic acid builds in the muscles. There are times when there are imbalances in the spinal fluids and it causes a kind of fuzziness or aching in the head. Would suggest that large quantities of water be taken on a daily basis. Would suggest the elimination of any caffeine products in the body. Would suggest elimination of any kind of chemical sweetener or chemical preservatives, a much more organic diet, fresh fruits and vegetables, organic meat. Less processed foods would be helpful. The more simple diet toward the macrobiotics would be very helpful and cause a cleansing in the body and would cause there to be more balance in the enzymes, the hormones, and the energy itself in the body the way it functions."* Because of the physical disorders, her body is aging very quickly, and suggestions were given for changing this.

She really wanted to know what was going on, and she received much more than she had imagined possible. For instance in addition to the description of mental and emotional disorders, the analysis very clearly connected specific ways of thinking to the physical disorders they feed: *"Being able to instill flexibility in the thinking, embracing the attitude that has been described, is most important in causing the spine to rejuvenate itself to become more flexible and usable. We see that this would aid then the nerves that feed the systems of the body, for it would open the channel through which the impulses do travel from the spinal cord."* This was particularly helpful for this woman because she wanted to learn and she was ready to respond to suggestions given.

The suggestion about her "casting off the cloak" was so clear in her mind that it was again, a very simple, a very clear image that she could hold in her mind and even do at times that enabled her to make the change. If she just told herself to quit feeling burdened or to cooperate, that wasn't the same. The full context of this idea was *"Would suggest that this can be changed by lifting the burden from her shoulders by imaging very clearly herself as being open and loving and embracing of what comes to her rather than being weighted down by it. In essence would suggest that this one use a mental image of throwing off a cloak of burden and opening her arms and embracing what is before her. This would give this one a place to initiate change and would lighten this one's attitude."* Casting off the cloak of burden was a crystal clear image that she really liked and it became her phrase to help her change the attitude that is harming her.

The Married Couple

The Husband

He came for his wife and for their marriage.

When they first came they were heavy. I mean they sat there and just didn't smile. The husband would look at the wife, taking his cues from her. After a while he would start lightening up a little then he would look at his wife and she wouldn't be smiling yet so he would go back to his frown. He was there for her and he wasn't going to change if she wasn't okay yet. His Health Analysis opened with *"This one is often troubled by others particularly those whom this one holds great affection for or whom this one relies upon in the life in some form and we see that this one uses this as a stimulus to avoid facing himself."* So his first challenge was realizing he could personally gain something through this weekend as well as help support his wife.

There was a clear suggestion to him to remember the things that he used to dream or think about when he was younger. The mentor asked him to remember those. He looked over at his wife and then looked back and said "I can't think of anything."

His wife said, "I want you to say them. Don't think that if you say them you are going to hurt me because it won't. Go ahead and say them. I want you to say them." He still didn't.

Finally she brought up a dream he has had for a long time, getting his Ph.D. He's getting close but still has his dissertation to write. As the weekend progressed he began to talk more and in the remembering he began to hear that he had used experiences in his life as excuses to keep him from finishing his dream. As he gained new perspective, he started smiling and laughing. It was as if his own burden was being lifted.

It was very difficult for him to talk. He was shaking at times when he was talking. It was tough. And you could tell in his voice and in his body how hard it was for him just to carry on a conversation with somebody. His analysis said, *"We see that this one is very inner in many ways and we see that much of what this one truly thinks and believes and wants is held very deep within himself. We see that it is not only kept from others but is often kept from himself as well and that by focusing on somebody else he can avoid really delving into himself."* He did open up and reveal a lot of himself. Before the close of the weekend, all the participants told him how much they had benefited by having him there, even before he opened his mouth. He made the weekend what it was just by him being there. He said if he used one word to describe his experience it would be challenge. He started out the weekend only for his wife, knowing the challenges she needed to meet. He realized the challenge in *his* life.

The fact that his wife was there really is going to be a benefit to him because they will be able to encourage each other to continue with it. And to remind each other of the content in their analysis. The weekend ended with a circle of love, the traditional closing for School of Metaphysics' classes and gatherings. At one point in the circle of love, one person turns to whomever is on their right and after saying their first name says, "I love you just because you are." The husband teared as he had the opportunity to express this to his wife. This was the beginning of following a suggestion his analysis had given: *"how to take action in the world."* The Health Analysis said, *"We see within the emotional system that this one is often times out of touch with his feelings. We see that this is purposeful because this one has very definite ideas about the emotions and what is proper and improper or what this one will allow and not allow. Would suggest that this is not to say that this is bad or that it is a difficulty, but it is a way that this one has learned to identify and to catalogue how this one reacts and to control his reactions. Would suggest that what is being addressed here is not a reaction to the world, but how to take action in the world. And this is an entirely different viewpoint of the emotions."* He was on his way to exploring new facets of himself, parts that would also enrich his marriage.

The mentor commented that it was very obvious how these two love each other. The husband came because he wanted to improve their marriage. Through the weekend the love they have for each other showed. They care. They really want the best for each other. It was really a beautiful thing to see, and added so much to the weekend for all the other participants. It became part of the healing energy generated through the weekend. Because of the intent and the personal enrichment each received through the weekend, their marriage was strengthened in unexpected ways.

The Wife

When she starts feeling like something is getting really hard to do she drags her feet, or wants to stop altogether. She says she does that all the time.

Even when she started reading her analysis to the others at the session she said, "This is really long, I just don't want to read it because it is just so long." Everyone just laughed saying, "There you're doing it, again." She said she does it with a lot of things. She said, "I do it with my job, my marriage, a lot of things in life." This weekend she became aware of the effect it has on others.

Her analysis suggested that she laugh. It also described ideas that helped everyone, *"...We see that meditation upon light is very important to this one. Would suggest this one would fill the Self with light in whatever way she knows. Whether it is through meditation or wearing light clothing, being in light places, turning on more lights where this one is. Light is very important to this one and can be a stimulus for a transformation in the way this one views life, for where there is light there can be seen what life has to offer. Where there is darkness nothing can be seen."*

In each group that comes together to create a session there are unifying factors, common needs and compatible desires which cannot be known until the session unfolds. This is how healing reveals itself. It is the miracle experienced by each one present.

With this group that factor was the denial of true desires or needs. Each one in some way or another was trying to avoid something and each used the session to muster the courage to face their own soul. This was simply and eloquently described in the intuitive reports:

"This one has much to offer but it is only through the action of giving that this will become apparent."

"Would suggest that this one become much more intrigued by answering the mysteries of life than merely being able to know that they exist."

"...as this one will begin to embrace the soul's urge for growth, this one will find a freedom that she has long sought and at times abandoned."

Before participants depart on Sunday they imagine what they are going to do to ensure they perpetuate the consciousness transformation that has been initiated. A guided imagery helps them to consciously use their imagination, setting into motion what will occur on Monday when they are back home, back at their jobs, back in the "real world" they have made for themselves.

Some imagine physical things. One said, "I'm going to go and finish the project I've been working on for two years. I'm going to finish that project." Another said, "I was really impressed with the meals. The quality of the meals and how they were served and the fellowship around the table and I'm going to start giving more attention to meals." Another said, "I'm going to go clean my room".

By holding the desired image and living that image others in their lives will be influenced just as much as they had been influenced by the old attitudes. It will not be an uphill climb where the familiar environment will try to steal away the new awareness or bury it in the past. They have the power. It requires much less energy to think positively than to think negatively. By cooperating with their true desires, they will become an attractive force, as they demonstrated throughout the weekend time and again. These experiences are now vital memories to draw upon for support, encouragement, and strength as they forge a new path in their continuing quest for wholeness and health.

Their *mental alarm* brings what they have learned into the present moment, wherever they are, whoever they are with, whatever they are doing. Psi awakening teaches an esoteric practice necessary for concentration. Identifying the distraction precedes the capacity to point the mind with desire. By having a mentor to assist in understanding and responding to their analyses, participants receive the best kind of health care. The introspective-interactive time has been well spent because now it can be applied in their daily life. They have everything they need to cause permanent change because they have already begun changing what is causing their greatest problem. Like a butterfly emerging from a cocoon, they have spent a weekend solely devoted to Self awareness and revelation, now they can freely emerge to beautify their environment and uplift the vibration of everyone they meet and everything they touch.

The best of religious philosophy and creative science unite to produce healing of mind, body, and spirit. Psi awakening initiates a means to continue pursuing lines of thinking and action that will perpetuate the healing beyond the confines of the weekend.

Once this challenge is met, participants can go on to another idea described in their analysis, mastering the next challenge until they achieve the wholeness and health that is their personal quest.

Part III

100 Years is but a Moment to the Soul

The natural healing force within each of us

is the greatest force in getting well.

> *– Hippocrates, Greek physician, 4th century B.C.*

It is part of the cure to want to be cured.

> *– Lucius Annaeus, Roman philosopher, 1st century*

It has been increasingly evident,

as pointed out by doctors everywhere,

that physical health is closely associated with,

and often dependent upon, spiritual health.

> *– Dr. Loring T. Swaim, former president*
> *American Rheumatism Association, 20th century*

Why Pain, Why Disease, "Why Me?"

John Clark has been facing death since he was fifteen. That was when he was diagnosed with juvenile onset diabetes and told he would need an artificial source of insulin in order to live.

A modern-day Angulimala, John has dealt with his demons all his life. Unlike Angulimala he has not taken the life of others, but he has in many ways stolen life from himself. Repeated self-indulgence has come at a high cost for John. He has faced death many times. He is now witnessing the effects of years of abuse, years of refusing to create positive change in himself and his life. His story is at times poignant, at other times infuriating, perhaps because we can so easily relate to it. Although diabetes may not be our "cross to bear" some other physical disorder is.

When disease enters your life you first want to restore wellness. You want to become whole again. If it's a virus you want it to be cleansed from your body. If it's diseased tissue you want it replaced by healthy, functioning tissue. If it's inner turmoil you want it resolved so the mind and heart can find peace. And most of us are like John, we want it right now. When it is not forthcoming, we determine our own destiny by how we fight or respond to change.

Ultimately, we discover that our desire to be healthy depends upon answering a question that arises in everyone's mind: "Why me?" Sometimes the question seems easy to answer. If you bring home a severe case of poison ivy from that beautiful weekend in the woods the answer to why readily comes. If you are the parent of an eight year old with a brain tumor the answers are not so easy to find. Because disease is so much a part of the human experience, what it brings to us is also similar. Yes, it can bring pain. It can also bring relief.

I've heard some people claim, in retrospect, "I needed to have that disease in my life." This is usually in the context not of the suffering endured but of what has come from facing the diseased condition. Families are reunited to battle an invader that threatens to take one of their own. People share what has long been withheld, forging bonds of friendship and love that laid fallow for years. Some cease self-destructive behaviors, replacing them with health-producing ones. Some inspire, teach, or aid others from their experiences.

I don't believe anyone *needs* to have disease in their life, yet when it arises I know there is a reason. That reason always centers around fighting change. By researching what causes health and wholeness, necessary prerequisites to fulfilling potential and cultivating genius, we have discovered etheric energy connections between the mind and body. In the course of our study we have isolated the misconceptions in the mind that produce malfunctions in the body. Beyond the consciousness implications of Dr. Kubler-Ross' five stages of dying, are specific patterns of thinking that organize energy in the mind and in the body. Ultimately, what we are seeing again and again is that disease is a physical manifestation of a type of thinking that is illustrative of what needs to change. Obviously we want the body to change when it is sick. We want it to be healthy. The truth is we must equally desire the mind to change, for until it does the illness will reappear.

Some see this as punishment. It is not. A life well-lived is the result of self-awareness and self-control. A life lived carelessly cannot manifest greatness but it will manifest a life that cares less. In the Western world of Christianity Jesus best described it "as you sow, so shall you reap." The concept is common sense, it is simple, and it is universal. When you plant an acorn, an oak tree grows. When you plant seeds of love, harmony grows, mind and body are strong. Plant seeds of self-condemnation, unworthiness grows, and your kidneys suffer. Indulge ideas of defensiveness and your immune system will weaken. Refuse to face facts and your ability to see with your eyes will decline. Each thought, whether positive or negative, creates an energy pattern that eventually is reflected in the physical life and body.

Disease indicates a karmic debt that needs to be paid. Because of its Eastern origins, many in the Western world jokingly dismiss the concept of karma. Having only a superfluous knowledge of the concept they fail to learn karma's relationship with Isaac Newton's Laws of Relativity. In its expanded context, karma denotes the workings – in the individual's soul and body – of the Universal Law of Cause and Effect. Karma is the means by which the soul matures for it enables us to understand what we cause. Intention causes Karma. Understanding relieves it. When there's the recognition of what the karmic debt is and the debt is paid there is a restoration to balance, what we call health or wholeness.

The typical response goes something like this, "Well I don't see how that can be true because I certainly didn't intend to get sick." Although a few may knowingly manufacture illness for their own motives most people do not. Yet who of us cannot recall an upset stomach that fortuitously kept us home from school on the day of a test we weren't prepared for, or a headache which gave us an excuse to go lie down thus escaping an unpleasant situation. There is no doubt that thought has energy. When that energy is intelligently directed it is a powerful creative element in our lives, fostering growth and causing healing.

The reality is that most diseases known to man, and all of the noncontagious diseases, are the result of specific ways intelligence and energy have been used. What exists in the imagination of the sculptor is revealed as he wields his chisel on stone. So it is with each of us. What exists in our imaginations is revealed as we use our will to fashion our lives. A disciplined imagination is the cornerstone for every good man has ever created. An undisciplined imagination, one filled with all manners of fear and doubt, is his greatest curse upon himself and his neighbor. This is illustrated in John's life.

John's story is an oxymoron, bitter and sweet. For almost twenty-five years he has been living on borrowed time and his series of Intuitive Health Analyses, which span a decade, reveal a startling history of awarenesses offered that were denied and opportunities presented that were refused. Amazingly, the analyses reveal how a treatable disease goes from bad to worse, revealing the mind's descent into destructive attitudes that lead to life-threatening conditions. They also show how at any time disease can be treated effectively through mental and physical disciplines that redirect what otherwise is a darkly predictable path to the end of life.

As part of his personal transformation John opens his life to us all in the hope that others may learn more quickly and more easily what it has taken him so long to realize. The following is his story, excerpted from the booklet *Vital Ingredient,* written by John's wife Dr. Laurel Clark.

John was a smart and active boy, full of energy and enthusiasm. Friendly and sociable, he made friends easily and wanted very much to be liked. Extremely talented, but highly undisciplined, he was the classic case of a child labeled by his teachers "great potential but needs to study. Is capable of much higher performance."

His greatest accomplishments occurred when he was directed by a strong coach, choir director or teacher. He excelled in sports, won wrestling trophies, played on football and basketball teams, and developed his beautiful tenor voice in church choirs. When he was diagnosed with diabetes at the age of 15, John denied the seriousness of the disease although secretly he started imagining the worst. He even said to himself (after being told of possible future complications), "When I lose my eyesight then I'll begin to take care of myself. For now I can eat what I want because I'm so athletic it won't matter."

And so he did. Ignoring sensible advice, he tested the limits of his endurance. He drank beer, smoked marijuana, ate sweets and fried foods, and injected insulin to counteract the effects of a rich, out-of-balance diet. His young body was strong, and the high level of physical activity helped to keep his blood sugar levels somewhat balanced. What John failed to admit was that the extreme swings from high to low were taking a toll on his body.

His mother and relatives prayed for him when he developed diabetes and counseled him to keep a positive attitude and trust in God. John never pursued seeking a reason for him developing the disease. It did not occur to him that this was a sign, or warning, or message, that there was something for him to learn from this experience.

Nor did he respond to the need for discipline demanded by diabetes: the need to pay attention to his diet, to eat at regular times, to monitor closely the amount of physical exercise and balance it with the amount of insulin. He continued to live as he always had, spontaneously, doing things at the spur of the moment without much planning or foresight.

In college when he was engaged in activities he liked, he gave himself to them and shone brilliantly. At other times he was undisciplined and lazy and managed to pass with minimal effort. After college, with a major in communications, John decided he wanted to be an actor so he moved to Chicago. During this time, John never really examined why he was living as he was. He became tired more easily. He was not always able to push himself to the physical limits that he had in the past. But still he did not relate this to his diabetes, nor think very deeply about why he even had the disease. It was just a circumstance in his life that he dealt with as he needed to.

Nearly fourteen years after first discovering that he had diabetes, John received his first Intuitive Health Analysis:

> *...we see within the mental system there is a great deal of frustration that this one is holding onto mentally. We see that much of this is the formation of this one's own ideas as to what this one needs to battle against concerning the environment. We see that there are many ways in which this one does try to escape this one's own responsibilities. We see that there is a battle which is occurring in that this one is not responding to what it is that this one does want to accomplish and does want to do. Would suggest that by making the environment and what this one considers to be the expectations of society a scapegoat for the Self, and the excuse as to why this one is frustrated with the lack of being able to achieve goals, there will continue to be the frustration that is spoken of. Would suggest that each day this one set out to do something that is solely for the Self....in initiating that, this one could see that there is the time if this one will cause it to be available for the Self. Would suggest also to this one to listen to the ways that this one uses such phrases as 'should, ought to, needs to, or has to' do. Would suggest that in this way this one is setting outside and away from the Self any freedom that this one has and likewise is setting aside from the Self the responsibility for the action on the part of the Self, therefore putting it in the hands of others. Would suggest that by doing something that this one wants to do each day, this will aid this one in understanding that is to the Self that responsibility does lie... [6-1-87-GBM]*

This analysis was helpful to John, because it brought to his attention the ways that he was keeping himself entrapped in limitations. He admitted to feeling like a victim and blaming his girlfriend for his failure to pursue his acting career. Prior to this, it had not occurred to him that *"responsibility"* meant much more than paying bills and taking care of physical needs. The analysis stimulated him to think more deeply about what *"responsibility to Self"* meant. A pattern began to emerge that John had yet to face: a need to understand himself as a spiritual being with a higher purpose for life than physical survival.

Would suggest that it would be important for this one to become honest in developing a worthiness as to this one's existence and a direction to be taken to fulfill this one's own purpose for existence.

This suggestion was offered to heal scarring that had occurred in the area of the liver. At this time, John had no awareness that there were any problems with his liver until he heard it in the analysis. Other physical effects of his "disordered" attitudes included sluggishness in the lymph system, the spleen, the small intestines, and the colon. Because he had no physical pain and no outward indication of problems in these areas, John ignored that part of the report. As he was to discover much later, he habitually waited for some kind of loss to motivate himself to change.

The changes he made in response to the analysis were primarily physical changes. He had yet to address the fundamental issues of his own Self worth and creating a deeper purpose for living.

A year later, John received another analysis. His primary concern was an injury he had received to his face; he had been struck by a baseball bat resulting in a massive bruise and black eye. The report said the healing was progressing and just needed time, so John was satisfied. He did not really understand, nor pay attention to a simple and profound statement that explained why it was taking so much time for the healing to take place:

There is somewhat of an attachment to the condition that exists. When there is no longer the need for the attachment, then the skin can be produced as this one would have it. This one tends to use particular conditions and holds onto them, even though they may be unpleasant, as reminders to the self to identify to identify those causes. (8-25-88-GBM-1C)

This analysis foreshadowed a gradual process of physical deterioration that eventually captured John's attention. It took him almost ten years to develop this awareness and to admit that his thoughts were causing his body to be as it was.

He asked about the condition of the diabetes and was told:

We see that there is a fluctuation in the activity as far as the pancreas is concerned. We see that as this one increases this one's reasons for identification with producing life within the self, this one can bring about changes here.

All John heard was that his pancreas wasn't dead. Traditional medical doctors had told him that diabetes meant an inactive pancreas. When he heard that his pancreas still had the ability to produce insulin, he was relieved but did not use that knowledge to face what he needed to change: the reasons for producing life within the self. He was still viewing his body as a machine, disconnected from his own thoughts and attitudes.

As a result, some of the physical conditions worsened. By November of 1988, (the next time John received an Intuitive Health Analysis), his pancreas was producing but not releasing insulin. This analysis echoed the one John received in June of 1987.

...We see that much of the conflict that this one is experiencing is a reorganization of this one's ideas of responsibility. We see that this one is attempting to change the ideas of responsibility as physical only, or being seen as burdensome to being more expanded in their outlook and in their influence or reaching effect. We see that this one has the ability to resolve these issues. This one has the knowledge, and the skill as well as the creativity to come to terms with who this one is and what this one desires. Would suggest that this one release doubt concerning this, and begin to move forward into the resolve that this one does have...

Again this analysis mentioned the need to focus upon desire and to express what he wanted. In fact, the analysis suggested that the mental cause for the diabetes was a need to understand himself as a creative being:

We see that much of this difficulty in the pancreas would be resolved as this one would learn to direct the creative ability purposefully. It is at times when this one fails to admit the purposes of the self and therefore create them actively that this one falls into feeling like he's being taken from or taking from others, falls into the difficulty in terms of the responsibility that has been described already, and this is what causes there to be imbalances in the pancreas itself. (11-1-88-BGR-7)

This passage is particularly significant, not just for John, but for many people in this day and age. Diabetes is one of the most common diseases in the United States and is becoming more prevalent in other countries as well. Why? It has been attributed to diet, lifestyle, genes. This analysis sheds some light on collective attitudes that have become more prevalent, thus increasing the incidence of diabetes. Many, many people question their purpose in life. Often, these people want to know what they will "get out of" a job or a marriage. We have become attached to physical success, physical possessions, acquisition of fame and fortune. The reason we have physical possessions and physical life itself is for us to create! A purposeful existence comes from giving ourSelves to our endeavors, knowing who we are and how to contribute to make the world a better place. As one becomes more creative and purposeful, the pancreas does its job effectively. When we take what we can get from life, the pancreas shuts down.

This would change as this one would become attached to understanding the experiences of the self rather than attached to the experiences for experience's sake.

John admitted (years later) that at the time he had this analysis, he heard the words but did not know how to put them into practice.

John's sixth analysis in 1992, showed a dramatic decline in his physical health. The attitudes were similar to those in previous analyses, but by this time (six years after his first health analysis) they had become more ingrained. The need for Self worth, for viewing himself as a spiritual being, for being motivated by a higher purpose, and to live rather than survive, were all addressed here. Because John had not changed these core attitudes, the effects on his body were more pronounced. The earlier analyses had said some of the problems were minor. In this one, it said the more he created a façade to cover up what he viewed as faults, "the farther and farther this one removes the self from the Truth and the ability to become whole." He was identifying more with being unhealthy, mentally, emotionally, and physically. This analysis noted breakdown in the capillaries, problems with the kidneys, and for the first time, signs of diabetic retinopathy (breaking of blood vessels in the back of the eye that can lead to blindness if left untreated.) Because John was not seeing himself clearly as a spiritual being with a higher purpose in life and because he was blinded to his true nature, his eyes were showing deterioration. The very first analysis John had noted a need for him to trust his perception; by this time his refusal to do so was reflected in some loss of physical vision.

When John heard this analysis, he could immediately link it to the facts in his life. He was having financial difficulties both in his own life and with the organization he directed. Rather than admitting it openly and asking for help or guidance, he tried to hide it, covering up mistakes in the checkbook and then becoming afraid someone would find out. Because his physical health was declining, John gave more and more attention to the needs of his body and removed more and more attention from the spiritual purpose for his existence. Some kind of counseling would have been of great benefit to him at this time, as he felt alone, trapped, and limited and this was all a product of his own thinking.

As all the analyses had noted, John's creative drive was unchanneled. He desired to be a loving, giving individual, helping other people and using his artistic and musical talents. But he had fallen into habits of pretending rather than imagining, being critical or sarcastic rather than genuinely entertaining, and fearful rather than creative. He could force himself into activity when his survival demanded it, but in so doing he was continually reacting to his environment rather than causing the life he was capable of living. Now, twenty years after the initial diagnosis of diabetes, his body was declining rapidly. This increased his fear. He knew he needed to do something fast; he could tell that his vision was getting worse, he had recurrent infections that would not heal, his nerves had suffered some damage and he had already lost feeling in his extremities. John still had difficulty admitting to himself and to other people that he had limitations; thus, many of the physical conditions worsened because he would not seek any kind of medical advice until he absolutely had to. He sought laser surgery to stop the bleeding in his eyes, and he began to see a chiropractor and Chinese herbalist for treatment of the diabetes. As John describes it, "I kept thinking I wasn't going to be able to get what I wanted. I was kind of desperate because at that point I was starting to have visual problems. I started to go to the Chinese herbalist because I was thinking I had to do something right then; I was getting worse quick. I didn't want to share that with anybody. I was doing things physically rather than attempting to do things mentally. Those Chinese herbs were a desperate attempt to fix my pancreas."

Again, it was pointed out that John needed to know himself as a spiritual being and to contemplate a deeper purpose for living. He was being more disciplined in a physical way. The attention he was giving to physical care had positive effects on his body, but in order for the healing to be complete it was essential that John also treat himSelf in a loving way. This included him embracing learning and creation as a way of life. Oftentimes, he was reckless or foolish, driving too fast, sleeping too little, picking at scabs until they became scars, forcing himself into action when he needed rest. He asked why he did such destructive things.

In part it is a result of apathy, but the apathy has arisen because this one has needed to learn the value of the will. This one has a very strong will. Because of this, this one has been indestructible. We see that this one has only recently recognized the force with which this one has tried again and again to prove his strength. We see that the destructiveness has arisen from this one wanting to eliminate weakness, to detach the self from it, to, in essence, destroy that which this one believed was weak. We see that this has come from a misunderstanding and a refusal to recognize the strength of this one's will to live. (4-17-93-BGC)

This is a most instructive lesson, especially for anyone who has a chronic illness. Western medical treatments often focus on eliminating disease or disorder: destroying cancer with chemotherapy, cutting out diseased organs with surgery and attempting to restore wholeness with drugs. Much of John's learning revolved around him accepting himself with all of his strength and weaknesses, all of his understandings and misunderstandings, all of his talents and all of his needs. Until he was willing to simply accept himself he kept trying to either deny the facts of his condition or force himself into being in a different place than he was.

...This was a turning point for John. When he first discovered that he had diabetes he tried to ignore it. Gradually, as his physical body became less and less strong, as he became more and more tired, as he experienced more and more parts of his body shutting down, he had to pay attention.

"I remember years before that, even when I was in high school, thinking about my eyes, and thinking I can do this [be irresponsible about taking care of myself] until my eyes start to go, and then I can change.

"Now I see that back in 1987 the liver was showing problems, and the kidneys, too, but I didn't even bother to look at that. I was in denial and didn't want to face facts. I didn't want to read *Diabetes Forecast*. I didn't want to talk to other people who were diabetics. I didn't want to admit to people that I was diabetic. I think I just thought I was indestructible, but never even admitted that until I heard about it in this analysis. I started realizing the fragility of my physical condition."

This denial showed up in an analysis two years later, in 1995. In the two years intervening John still tried to force healing to occur, holding on to doubt and relying on willfulness to move him to action. Put simply, John was afraid to change. He was attached to things as they were, even though they were often unpleasant. The physical changes that had started in 1993 were slowing down, and his body was again showing the deterioration that had been taking place for years now.

> *The pancreas cannot be forced to change physically, therefore this one must adjust in the mental and emotional systems. This one must learn how to initiate and to sustain motion. This one must learn how to surrender. (1-18-94-BGC-7)*

John knew that he had to make some mental changes because he knew the physical things weren't working so well any more.

Within six months, John awoke one day and found that he could hardly see out of his right eye. He knew that his eyes had gotten progressively worse since he first noticed blurriness in 1990, but this still came as a shock. At the insistence of his wife he went to an eye doctor who told him that he needed immediate surgery to arrest further damage, although much of the damage that had already occurred was irreversible. Imagining the worst, John got another health analysis:

> *We see denial within this one. We see that for a long period of time this one has refused to face facts about the self. We see that as a result of this, this one is continually in fear that this one will find out something that this one is ill-equipped to handle. As a result of this, this one continually sets up conditions and circumstances in which this one does produce the results of this one's fears.*
>
> *Would suggest to this one that there is a need for this one to build a desire for awareness. We see that there is a need for this one to form an*

image of the benefits that will be derived from this one knowing what is within the self and from knowing what is without the self, for we see that until this one does have awareness, this one will have very little basis to create from or to create with. (5-25-95-LJC-1M)

John knew that he was afraid, particularly because the near complete loss of eyesight in his right eye and partial loss of sight in the left eye meant that he could not drive. His whole sense of identity had been crumbling and now suffered a complete crash.

A series of choices and circumstances further amplified John's fear. He had major surgery done on the right eye. Because of the physical deterioration and increasing weakness of his body, including the lymph system, he developed an infection in the eye where the incision had been made. For a period of time John experienced extreme headaches, then further complications from the surgery resulted in a total loss of sight in his right eye.

(Three months later) he had another episode of bleeding in the back of his eye. As he described it, "everything was fuzzy; I could not focus." Since he was completely dependent on one eye for sight, the additional loss of vision was terrifying. The doctor said that the new bleeding and scar tissue was pulling the retina away from his eye. He said that John had no choice; if he did not have surgery he would become totally blind in six months to a year because the scar tissue would pull the retina completely away from his eye.

He sought a second opinion and the second doctor also recommended surgery since the benefits of surgery outweighed the risks.

This was on Thursday. As John describes it, "The bottom line was that I was scared, nervous, and wanted to be with people over the weekend. So it happened, my miracle weekend! The news of my upcoming surgery traveled to the National Headquarters of the School of Metaphysics, then to another teachers meeting in Kansas City. When I spoke with my wife, she told me that the college students and the teachers at the Kansas City meeting wanted to do healing on me; would I give permission? I responded yes! At the Dallas meeting Dr. Sheila Benjamin informed me she would do 'hands on healing' before the Interfaith Church of Metaphysics service if I requested it. I did. I also participated in a healing class Sunday evening and received more healing. I called my mother and told her of the upcoming surgery and asked for her prayers. She called her friends and my brothers and sisters who all prayed for me.

"Monday morning my wife and I set out for St. Louis. As I went through the routine of testing the eyes, there was a drastic difference in the left eye. On Thursday, all I could read was the giant "E" on the eye chart. On Monday I could read several lines farther down, and I could focus. The doctor's assistant said my vision had improved from 20-300 to 20-30 from last Thursday. 'I'm just a student,' she said, 'but I think the doctor may not do surgery.' When the doctor came in, he examined my left eye, re-examined it and repeated three times, 'something has changed'. He said that something must have changed over the weekend because the scar tissue that had been pulling the eye from the retina had been dislodged or dissolved. It was no longer there. He then advised me not to have the major operation, and to let him do laser treatment instead. This would stop the bleeding and be much safer than a major operation requiring an incision and general anesthesia.

"What had happened? What had occurred? My eye had improved in three days. I began to put the pieces together: went to teachers meeting, was in a healing environment with other teachers and metaphysicians, received hands-on healing from Doctor Sheila, as well as being healed by the teachers in Dallas, Kansas City, the healing classes in Springfield and at the college, and healing prayer from my mother and family. Yes, I must be receptive to healing. Yes! I asked for healing. I prayed for healing. I meditated for answers to the question of surgery or not. My quest for understanding has a vital ingredient, which is to ask. Ask for courage, ask for love, receive truth."

You might think that this is the end of the story, a happy, hopeful, positive ending to a tumultuous journey. John was receptive to healing because he was scared. He was afraid that this surgery might turn out as the previous one had. If he lost the vision in the left eye he would have no eyesight at all. Remember all of those analyses that counseled him to focus on desire? In this situation he concentrated his attention completely on the desire for an alternative to the surgery, and he received what he asked for! But once the crisis was over, John's doubts crept back in. He even began to doubt that the miracle he experienced was real. He rationalized that the first doctor had misdiagnosed his condition rather than continue to build upon belief in the power of the mind to cause miraculous healing. Although he did not admit it, accepting the miracle of his healing meant that he was responsible for a new way of thinking.

Although it was too late for John to change the past, he could live now and needed to live now. For reasons oftentimes unknown to his conscious mind, his soul still wanted to use this physical body even with its limitations and areas of degeneration. This analysis described the disorders in the liver, kidneys, gallbladder, and pancreas that had been there for awhile, and continuing deterioration in the nervous system and circulatory system. The eyes showed scarring and blood vessel proliferation, and when John asked how to heal the eyes, the report said:

> *In order for there to be change in this area, this one does need to decide that this one wants to see what is present within the self and what is present around the self and as long as this one dwells in the past and avoids facing what is truth in the present, this condition will continue.*

By this time, John did admit that in order to cause physical changes that would become permanent, he needed to change his ways of thinking. He had tried so many different physical remedies and treatments, had tried different doctors and healers, had listened to advice from many well-meaning friends and relatives. Every time he found a treatment that produced temporary change in his body, he was relieved, but soon afterwards his body would begin its destructive course once again. This time, he asked what changes to cause mentally in order to produce permanent healing:

> *Would suggest to this one that this one does need to admit responsibility for what has occurred within the Self and within the life. Would suggest that this one cease viewing this as blame or condemnation, for we see that as long as this one views this as blame, this one does avoid facing the truth. Would suggest that this one create an attitude of discovery and create love for the self and for this one's ability to learn and to give this one's full attention to how this can occur and what this one wants to occur in the present. ... True responsibility is this one's power to create based upon the choices that this one has made and does make.*

When John heard this, he says "I still wasn't willing to look at what mental state I was in totally or fully accept that it was a place where I could learn or discover. I'd heard it intellectually but it didn't sink in. I didn't even look at my high blood sugar levels as a place of endangerment. I wasn't very diligent about what I ate or keeping my blood sugars down. I wasn't willing to face responsibility to accept a new way of thinking as the way to heal. I was still blaming, I was still condemning myself and blaming others. I wasn't willing to say, this is a great lesson for my soul. I was still expecting acupuncture, Chinese herbs, enzymes, all that stuff was somehow going to pull me through. I did not yet admit the big part that has to be done has got to be from me."

That winter John had a series of episodes during which his legs started to cramp, then spasm, until he could not even support his weight on them. He started doing acupuncture treatments and taking additional minerals which helped some, but he still experienced these convulsions from time to time. Twice during this time he blacked out for a brief period of time, finding out after the fact that his blood sugar levels had been extremely high. He did not relate the leg cramping and the high blood sugar reactions to each other at the time.

Then, in July, he was awakened from sleep by his legs twitching convulsively. Three times in a row he was rendered unconscious by seizures. He was rushed to the hospital and placed in intensive care. The doctors thought perhaps he was epileptic, since the seizures had the classical symptoms of grand mal epilepsy. A battery of tests including an MRI and EEG showed nothing, and the doctors were at a loss to discover the cause for the seizures. They insisted that John take Dilantin, an anti-seizure medication. John was not eager to take more medication. In the past year he had been put on three different blood pressure medications, diuretics, countless antibiotics, and still took insulin twice a day. The attending doctor would not release John from the hospital until he took the Dilantin so John did, but he did not like the effects of it at all. It affected his equilibrium and his thinking, making him foggy and unsettled.

The hospital stay was a big warning signal for John to take command of himself. John says, "How much more did I have to hear to take a step toward loving myself? I'm glad I made the choice to go into the hospital, because I think that ultimately the inactivity gave me an opportunity to sit there and think about what I was really doing. What did I want to do? I was stimulated to think, am I just trying to give up here?"

All of the tests, all of the technology, all of the medical books and medical knowledge had come up with a big "zero" in terms of identifying the cause for the seizures John experienced. He got a health analysis to understand what was going on. This, his thirteenth analysis, pinpointed what was going on in his thinking and how it affected him physically:

We see extreme tension in the mental system at the present time. We see that this is revolving around immediacy and reactions to stimuli that have occurred. We see that there is a great deal of extremes that this one is experiencing between turmoil and submission. We see that in order for this one to think more clearly and in order for this one to be able to pursue lines of thought and creative thought which would be of benefit to the Self, there needs to be a calming that would occur in the mental system. There needs to be a focus which this one can direct the energies toward and there needs to be the alertness of this one's willingness to contemplate. We see that this one is aware of the means by which these can be procured. We see that there is a need for this one to recognize the capability of the Self of accomplishing these.

We see within the mental system that there is attachment. The attachment is deep, and it is very strong. We see it has been practiced over a prolonged period of time. We see that it is toward anything of the physical. We see that this one has made a pattern of life in how this one is attached to how things appear to others, how things exist in regard to the environment outwardly rather than there being any sense of inward compass or means by which this one would direct the Self. We see that this has caused there to be severe limitations in this one's mental, emotional, and physical systems and we see that it has in effect produced the kind of existence that this one is in such turmoil concerning. We see that this one needs to become freer in the willingness to cultivate a connection with a sense of conscience. We see that this one's attachment to the physical has led this one to a point where it is more and more difficult for this one to deny the sense of inward environment. In essence this one is more and more feeling forced to turn inward. Would suggest that it would aid this one to be willing to surrender to the condition. This is not to say to give up anything, it is to say to be willing to open the Self completely to what is Truth and to merely direct the attention inwardly as much as this one can.

This suggestion to turn inward made perfect sense to John. Being in the hospital for five days, he did explore and examine his thoughts much more deeply than he had previously. There were no distractions and he had a great deal of time to simply sit and think. It was becoming clear to him why his physical senses were shutting down. He could relate to the idea of force, and now he was being forced to turn inward because he had been undisciplined in causing it. Why had he been so stubborn in refusing to do this earlier?

We see that this one has feared the inner parts of the Self and has imagined fears over such a prolonged period of time that this one has not had the desire to reach inwardly and has held on therefore the more tightly to those things of the physical, but we see that this one has not understood the nature of the physical existence and therefore this one is experiencing what are considered limitations that do stimulate this understanding within this one. Would suggest that this one still has volition, therefore there are many choices that this one can make and there are many choices that this one needs to make. Would suggest that this one begin by attaining the calmness that has been stated and by being willing to transfer the attachment to the inner Self rather than feel that he must give it up. Would suggest that this one also admit that the imagined fears that he has built over a prolonged period of time are a product of his imagination and therefore can be changed in a like manner. The worst that this one can think and can be is what this one has already manifested. It is not something that is unknown to this one.

John was ready, finally, to hear the suggestion to use his imagination productively. He contemplated the idea of surrender and used it. As a child he had been taught to pray but it had been years since he had made that a part of his life, and after hearing this analysis he reawakened his connection with God.

"I have had so many analyses before, but the biggest difference is that I've taken this analysis in. I haven't really dwelled on the physical stuff. It's there, but I've been focusing on what I can do with the mental and emotional direction from this analysis, and the physical stuff I've just simplified. In the other analyses, I heard the words but I didn't have a clue as to what to do about it. Here, I had a clue what to do. I understood what it said about being mentally tense and experiencing turmoil between tension and submission. Before, I looked at surrender as giving up, as weakness. Now I saw submitting being to surrender to the condition, a place of strength, a place where I could recover, and respond and be responsible. At first I thought I had no choice, [because everything was shutting down anyway] but once I started to do it I realized I did have choices! I was able to do it. I was able to respond and be responsible."

In 1996, John received another analysis. The information was not new. The difference was that John responded differently. "I've had those times where I felt like I was incapable so I had to stop and look for a solution, clear my mind, and where I needed help, to ask for it. The analysis talked about a sense of inward compass, and I wanted to find that inner compass, I wanted to get in touch with it. It really stimulated me to do every day what I had avoided and denied, going inward. I was willing to listen and I wanted to discipline my mind to listen for inner guidance every day...I finally understood surrender. In surrendering I was discovering, I was actually using what I had to offer in the situation rather than thinking I was being taken from by not being able to do certain things.

"In learning about diabetes, in learning how to control and direct my life, and the insulin, and eating, and all the factors of taking care of myself physically, it would lead to opportunities for me to give beyond just myself, which is what I want to do. Like, to be a teacher, to learn how to do all the things I'm going to learn to do without vision. Even if my body heals and I can see again I can be like my mobility teacher and teach people. It wouldn't be like I would be doing it for nil, or giving up because I was on a way of no return. Teaching people ... I was inspired by being in the hospital by what these people did by coming around and teaching me how to direct eating habits and choices. All these situations would lead to many areas that would be a place for me to give and teach and serve and to help others as well as myself. I hadn't seen that before.

"Why did I finally pay attention? I'm not sure. I think it was the whole scenario of events that happened. I had three seizures. That scared me. I went into the hospital. I felt really weak. The test showed my kidneys were failing, a third of my liver was gone and not working, the high blood pressure was a real risk of stroke, my eyes were going. I mean, you name it, my physical body was not there for me in every way. I was humbled by admitting where I was. Everything about my existence was slipping away.

"The physical part of the analysis shocked me. In just about every analysis prior to this one it talked about liver deterioration, but this one said that part of the liver was dead. I thought, my God! I had no idea it was that bad. It alarmed me, the seriousness of this. I knew that all this time I had been ignoring it, and I couldn't ignore it any more. I felt very determined, scared but determined. When I heard that it was caused by the refusal to become cognizant of anything that is not physical I thought , 'I have been totally oblivious to just how physical I was being, and it's killing me!' All of a sudden it just clicked about what really was the source of my existence. It wasn't my body! I needed a body. My soul needed a vehicle. And I also realized, if I'm still here, then my soul still wants to learn with this vehicle. So I decided that I want to give my soul some attention."

In the months following, John exercised much more care and discipline than he had in all the years since he had become diabetic. On a physical level, he learned more about how to adjust his insulin dosage and was more regular in testing his blood sugar levels. He paid closer attention to his diet. He had decided not to take Dilantin and instead used the suggestion to sound the two musical notes when he felt a seizure coming on, which proved to be effective in most cases. Spiritually, he continued to meditate and pray daily, and to listen to the inspirational and motivational tapes. He also started psi counseling to help him uncover and change the long standing habits that had kept him so engrossed in limitations. As a result, his condition started improving, not dramatically (as had occurred with the miraculous healing of his eye) but gradually.

The series of Intuitive Health Analyses John has had over a ten-year period show why his body has not healed despite the many different physical treatments he has tried. He has used Western medical methods — insulin, surgery, high blood pressure medications, antibiotics. He has used nutritional supplements — vitamins, minerals, enzymes, vegetarian diets, wheat grass juice, flax seed oil, aloe vera juice, colloidal silver, and more. He has tried alternative treatments — chelation therapy, acupuncture, liquid oxygen, Chinese herbs, colonic irrigation, chiropractic. These are just some of the ways he has tried to make his body keep running. Most of them have worked for a period of time to produce temporary physical improvement. But all of them, sooner or later, either ceased to interest John after the newness wore off, or ceased to work. His body simply adjusted to the new substances or treatments and followed the direction of his thinking.

John's analyses over the years showed a pattern which is revealed in the key words that repeat time after time: desire, purpose, imagination, worthiness, belief in Self, creative power. These are the karmic issues John has yet to face. When he focuses on what he loves, on who he is and how he can most genuinely give who he is to help other people, he is the most at peace and his body begins to heal. When he falls into old habit patterns of thinking of himself as worthless, he becomes selfish, holding back and becoming engrossed in identifying who he is according to his physical appearance, state of his physical body or the physical conditions in his life. Then he gets scared, because his physical body does not have the stamina it once had, he no longer has the use of his eyes, and he cannot do what he was once capable of doing physically. The analyses have pointed out that John has been motivated by fear. When he thinks he is losing something or when he has, in fact, lost something, then he is motivated to action. But clearly this kind of motivation is temporary. As soon as the crisis passes, he takes for granted what he has and waits for another crisis to spur him to action. His vast potential can only be channeled with regular, consistent discipline and he continues to discover that when he is disciplined change occurs.

I have often asked myself, why is John still alive? He has had so many near-death experiences and has lived so recklessly, it would have been very easy for him to die many times. But something keeps him going. Something within him urges him to stay here, in this physical body, this physical plane, this physical existence, this lifetime. What does his soul want?

The poet Kahlil Gibran said, "pain is the breaking of the shell that enclosed your understanding." Perhaps for some people it is only when they are in pain that they recognize what they are missing. If you don't know that you have something, how can you use it? Maybe for John the whole process of disease is a way for him to discover buried treasure — the treasure of his own understandings that he has taken for granted. There are lessons that John is learning that he did not learn when he had the full use of his body. Most of his life he has done things at the last minute, and now he cannot so easily procrastinate. Since he cannot drive, he must plan ahead to arrange bus rides. When he was younger, he made it through school without learning to concentrate; thus, he never discovered the full extent of his intelligence. Now, he must give attention to simple tasks like getting dressed or preparing a meal and can no longer get by with scattering his attention. To read, he must concentrate and immerse himself completely in what he is analysis using special magnifying lenses. He has to draw upon his resources in more creative ways and communication has become a necessity. He is trusting his intuitive perception to a greater extent, relying on telepathy and clairvoyance when he cannot see who is in the room.

Perhaps his greatest lesson right now is that he is a soul, not a body. This is a challenge. In high school he was voted "best body" and received acclaim for his athletic prowess. He used to make a living by modeling. He often searched for self worth through girlfriends; if women thought he was attractive he could believe that he had some value. He is still handsome, but his real beauty comes from within, when he is giving and sharing who he is. He is gradually discovering that the physical body he has been so attached to is not the same as it was twenty years ago. Ultimately, everyone must come to this realization, but it is not always a constant reminder that we live with every day. For John, daily he must face the fact that he is not his body. Daily he must nurture himself and live with discipline to cause his body to function.

I feel certain that when John has learned all he wants from this condition he will either heal or leave his mortal frame. For now, his life holds a message for anyone who wants to learn. The mind is tremendously powerful, and it is in our hands to determine the quality of our existence. We can live creatively, producing health, or we can deny the very reason for existence, and cause the body to wear out. The physical world has its limits, and so do physical treatments. They will work for awhile, but eventually restrictive attitudes cause physical breakdown. To go beyond survival, we must nurture the spirit. Every day holds opportunities to learn, to become better, wiser, more loving, more disciplined, more whole. As we learn, as we love, as we create, we have life.*

* Excerpted from *Vital Ingredient* by Dr. Laurel Clark. SOM Publishing, © 1998

What's Killing Americans?

John's story could be anyone's.

He has had the power to change the course of his life for years, but he has repeatedly forfeited that dominion. In the end, what John has learned from his choices will be what is carried by his soul into the afterlife. Yet, how very different his life could have been and still can be, if only he is willing to see things differently, to dream new dreams, to stop fighting life and start living it with dignity and integrity.

John's life is an allegory for us all. A lesson we can learn that begins by asking ourselves, "Do I embrace change in my life? Am I actively fostering admirable characteristics in myself? Am I consistently aiming to nurture productive traits and eliminate negative ones?" John's story reminds us that life is what we make it. We are our own creation.

Most people are like John. They are decent people with a sound upbringing, good stock, but they do not continue to learn throughout their lives. Gleaning understanding from life experience is essential for the growth of the soul. When we fight change we are refusing the lesson before us. Unless *we* change the lesson is force-fed to us. We describe it as failing a course, losing a job, getting a divorce. For the most part people stop learning when formal schooling ends, somewhere in early adulthood, and it is only a matter of time until it begins showing. For some, like John, disease comes early. For others it takes decades. The cost can be measured not only in money but in the waste of human potential trapped in diseased minds and bodies.

By examining the predominant diseases which rob people of life we can begin to identify the changes our society needs to make. This can mean the difference between people of good will who invest time, energy, and money in their community to make it a better place for everyone to live, and people who carry weapons and live behind security fences because they live in fear of one another due to violence, murder, and thievery. Society is comprised of many individuals desiring to live together. Using applied metaphysics we can pinpoint the cause of what ails us, indeed what kills us. By isolating the causal consciousness we can change individually and collectively to promote a healthier society. Now. Without large financial investment. Without government intervention.

Let's examine the primary causes of death in the United States in the latter 1990's. According to the U.S. Department of Health, the ten leading causes of death are:

1)   heart disease

2)   malignant growths

3)   cerebrum, blood vessel diseases

4)   unintentional injuries, including motor vehicle accidents

5)   chronic lung diseases

6)   pneumonia and influenza

7)   diabetes

8)   suicide

9)   human immunodeficiency virus

10) homicide

The School of Metaphysics exists to help accelerate evolutionary progress. We are invested in developing mankind's potential through personal excellence. This is why our research is centered upon *how* learning occurs, be it reasoning in the conscious mind, intuition in the subconscious mind, or realization in the superconscious mind. This focus has enabled us to explore reality from an unlimited point of view, seeing the progressive element in whatever is before us. We leave the traditional educational model of acquiring worldly knowledge to those who are expert in that area. We are constructing a new wholistic model based on mankind's need to know how learning transpires, how consciousness works. This is not a new field. It has been visited by the most innovative and profound thinkers throughout time, but it is one that is ready to be

The quest for self-knowledge has always been present in the individual. This has led to the type of mass communication of information available today. What is different today is the yearning for self-realization. This has been evidenced in greater numbers of people in our own time than ever before. So we are prepared to hear the truth. We can face the knowledge that we fight change and therefore make our own lives harsh. We can put to use the knowledge that we can put our minds into directive action manifesting our highly valued dreams. We are prepared to hear alternatives. We want to know what happens before birth, after death, and everything in between.

People are no longer willing to wait until death, or even near-death experiences, to attain peace of mind. In our daily lives, enhancing understanding brings greater peace. The more we understand ourselves – our motivations, our desires, our capacities, our origin, our destiny – the more we understand our Maker and our neighbor. This quality of understanding enables us to live with one another peaceably. These conclusions are based upon Universal Laws and Truths. These are not manmade laws. These laws exist beyond, and are the causal principles for, science's natural laws.

The physical body only exists when a soul is committed to using it for learning. To one familiar with the mental attitudes causing and promoting these disorders, these diseases that rape our bodies give an insightful look at the consciousness of our country as we approach the new millennium. Drawing upon thousands of Health Analyses which identify the mental cause of physical disorders and upon Dr. Daniel R. Condron's research recorded in the book *Permanent Healing,* these are the thought patterns, in brief, that initiate the diseases that most frequently terminate physical life:

1) Misuse or misunderstanding of responsibility; false ideas of responsibility or fearing it

2) Hatred of self

3) Misuse or incomplete use of thinking

4) Inattention to what is at hand

5) Thinking one's desires will not be fulfilled and blaming others for this; fearing a loss of freedom

6) Fear of desires not being fulfilled. Hesitation and indecision.

7) Refusing to give, deliberately withholding the self from others

8) Refusal to learn and cause change

9) Defensiveness caused by insecurity in identity; feeling power-less

10) Disrespect for life; refusal to control self's thoughts and emotions

These are negative attitudes. Unattractive at best and destructive at worst, they erode what is good in man, marring the beauty of life. They wound, scar, and eventually destroy. Negativity does effect others, even drawing to it those of like or compatible minds. But most important to realize is negative patterns of thinking are like a boomerang; they always return to their sender.

Viewing the list of "killers" as patterns of thinking sheds light upon the problems of modern society. We can begin to recognize these destroyers of life and liberty as individual dis-eases that are manageable, one person at a time. Automobile wrecks and murder are obviously societal ills. They potentially affect all our lives, disrupting them in every way from defiling our sense of personal security to consuming billions of dollars. This is also true of the other eight killers on the list.

Heart disease, cancer, and the rest become societal ills by their sheer numbers. But more than this, they indicate shared patterns of thinking that destroy the quality of life for the person who indulges in them and for everyone around him. It is not hard to find statistics about how illness affects us. From the outrageous costs of medical care and insurance to business absenteeism and faulty products to legally drugged public transportation drivers, individual disease and the ways we seek treatment affect all of us in very personal ways. Let's examine them more closely.

1)   Heart Disease

Symbolically speaking when someone says, "Have a heart" they are talking about kindness. They are urging us to give more than we presently are, to respond beyond what we have previously. When something "breaks our heart" we are figuratively describing the sorrow that accompanies something we experience but do not understand thereby feeling ill-equipped to respond.

Heart disease arises in those who have difficulty responding to life. Sometimes they are the kind of person who tries to compete with others and always finds himself lacking. From the young boy who can never be his big brother to the person who thinks he has to come up with a more expensive car than his neighbors, heart disease erupts in people who are pretending to be something they are not.

Such a person's life is not a reflection of his own values, but of those of others. The conditions in his life are not a manifestation of what he desires but what a spouse, employer, children, or friends want. Such a one is faking life because he isn't where he aspires to be. These attitudes distort the natural ability to respond to learning in life. The energy patterns they produce adversely affect the circulatory system function causing anything from the high blood pressure of "carrying the burdens of the world on your shoulders" to a heart attack from trying to "keep up with the Jones". All are a manifestation of a misplaced sense of responsibility.

"Having a heart" will empower you to respond in new, better, more fulfilling and joyous ways. Give up fighting change and accept, accept, accept! Through acceptance you can extend your ability to respond to the people and situations in your life. Responding brings a new attitude about the meaning of life. In time you will realize responsibility *is* freedom. The freedom to live, to love, to grow.

2)   Malignant Growths

Ask anyone how they don't want to die and nine times out of ten they will say "cancer." Cancer is the great fear of our society. And rightfully so if you consider the thought pattern supporting the disease is hatred. Hatred of self. Hatred of the self in relationship to others. A well-known black singer, who hated the fact that he could not or did not speak out against injustice, dies of throat cancer. A well-loved television star who hated that he was ostracized by others because of his religion dies of pancreatic cancer. A comedian who hated how she was treated as a woman often wishing her life was different dies of ovarian cancer. The preacher's wife who never had anything bad to say about anybody dies of cancer of the colon. Silently reinforcing resentments and grudges against the self, or others, breeds the normal cells that suddenly turn upon themselves in an explosion of growth, characteristic of cancer cells. Where the cancer begins is not chance. It too is the result of pattern of thinking that erodes the vitality and function of that particular system or organ.

Each person with cancer bears their hatred without fanfare and often without complaint. They do not dwell on the source of their irreparable wound but it is constantly with them, eating away at everything they think, say, or do. Others may know what eats at them, others may even understand it but the person with cancer does not. For them it is a wound that does not heal. The thinking pattern often begins with anger which is never resolved, never understood. It seethes and grows, festering into the hatred that fuels itself poisoning happiness and ultimately destroying its creator.

Giving is paramount for cancer recovery. In the action of (for)giving peace can be found. Loving life without reservation, unconditionally, even when at first you do not understand something, will begin a new, productive energy flow that will replace the old configuration.

3)   Cerebrum, Blood Vessel Diseases

The brain is an organ of the body. Intricate in its design, man cannot replicate it. Amazing in its function, man utilizes only a small portion of its potential.

Man's spirit exists before, during, and after the physical shell we call the body. It makes itself known in the conscious mind and outer personality. The brain is not the source of who man is any more than it is the source of information. The brain is like a computer with all the potential wiring for memory. The spirit, the mind, is the intelligence that turns the computer-brain on and utilizes it for investigation, communication, creativity, and learning. The brain enables spirit to synthesize what the body experiences:

what it sees, hears, tastes, touches, smells.

When we are mentally absent from life, withdrawing from life's challenges, we misuse our intelligence and will. Our skills begin to rust. We don't remember as well as we used to. We can't think straight. We're slower than we used to be. We are no longer exercising our thinking processes completely. We no longer act in life, reaching for learning. Now we react to life, repeating ourselves, weakening our capacity to respond to what life brings. We cease thinking and allow emotional reactions to determine our choices. We no longer feel wanted or needed by others. We feel different from others. This kind of thinking adversely affects the workings of the brain. Disorders ranging from stroke to senility begin to manifest themselves.

To rebuild sound thinking patterns, exercise thinking every day. Read mysteries and solve them. Work math problems instead of using a calculator. Make a new friend. Practice a concentration exercise daily. Set goals for a year from now, ten years, fifty years. Learn something you've wanted to know how to do since you were ten years old. Teach a child something your parents taught you that you still use every day. Rekindle an old friendship. Write letters, songs, novels, lists of things to do. Remember your dreams, write them down, and learn to interpret their meaning. Meditate everyday, it is what fuels your spirit. Volunteer your services. Smell the flowers, taste the fruit off a tree, touch the fur of a kitten. You are capable of so many good things, make sure you are doing at least one of them at all times.

4) Unintentional Injuries, including motor vehicle accidents

I remember reading statistics on what causes car accidents. The reason that surpassed all others is inattentiveness. Whether the result of drinking alcohol, the racing ego of an adolescent, or the phone conversation the person is attempting to pursue while also driving, scattered attention disperses the mind's perceptive capacity delaying commands to the body. What an attentive driver can safely respond to the distracted driver does not even see.

With any unintentional injury, the causal pattern of thinking is ignoring what is at hand. Refusing to face and respond to facts causes people to "accidentally" misjudge time and distance. They take the wrong medicine, miss a step, take unnecessary risks.

Keep in mind, if running a red light because you're in a hurry because you're late results in a car wreck, it was no accident. You broke the law, the agreements that enable us to live together. You were pushing it, chancing danger, and allowing an emotionally-tinged imagination to overrule your reasoning capacity to face the facts.

The cure for inattentiveness? It is something we Westerners are very poor at: live in the now. Contemplate the concept that the only moment you possess is right now. Now is the only time you can be, do, act, say, think, want, will, anything. Harness the power of your mind by focusing your attention to a single point. You can hone this ability into a skill with daily practice of concentration. As the skill builds it becomes natural to apply it in everyday situations.

5)   *Chronic Lung Diseases*

I grew up when information about the effects of smoking tobacco was just beginning to become public. In the '70's I saw an obvious dilemma arising concerning specifically the link between smoking and lung disease. It seems true that people who intentionally pollute their respiratory systems by inhaling smoke place enormous stress upon the body, expecting it to somehow rid itself of the poisons they voluntarily feed it daily. The common belief is the body cannot get rid of the toxins and over time they eventually build up promoting emphysema and cancer and all manners of chronic lung disease. For thousands of Americans this is true.

The dilemma comes when you consider the millions of people who smoke without suffering from problems and who die of other causes not related to their daily habit. In other words it happens to some but not to others. My question was "why?" It was answered not in the outer environment, where the dangers of smoking in the spacious outdoors of Montana pale in comparison to living in the suffocating air of Denver, Los Angeles, or New York City, but rather in the inner environment.

People who manifest chronic lung problems, from repeated chest colds as a child to allergies as a teenager and adult to chronic lung diseases of the latter years share a common way of thinking. They feel a loss of freedom of expression. A child must be quiet because a new sibling has joined the household. An adolescent finds her plans are thwarted by disciplining parents. A man thinks he can't say what he wants to say at work because he imagines he might lose his job. A woman feels she must think and act like a man to get where she wants to be in the corporate world. The classical henpecked husband realizes he never has finished his own sentences. In every case these people believe their desires will not be fulfilled, and they blame others for it. That is the thought pattern producing weakness in the respiratory system.

Expressing yourself is not making a pest, nuisance, or jackass of yourself. Expressing yourself is being aggressive, taking action upon your ideas and dreams. Create what you desire in life, don't wait for someone else to bring it to you on a silver platter. Exercise your free will to create what you want when you want it. You will soon realize that true freedom is the capacity to direct your attitude. That is the true control in life, you determining your attitude, not the people or situations around you.

6)   *Pneumonia and Influenza*

This killer is somewhat misleading. It appears on the list not for its inherent lethal nature but because it is enabled by conventional medicine. Many terminally ill hospital patients do not want to die from the disease that assails them. Nor are they allowed to by well-meaning physicians. They are kept alive by drugs and machines that postpone death from its primary cause. The hesitation – "I want to live but not like this", "I don't want to die but it has to be better than this" – is a symptom of Dr. Kubler-Ross's bargaining stage. By the time depression sets in the body is so ravaged by disease and the treatments meant to control it that pneumonia enters as a means for an already compromised bodily system to die. This is why pneumonia and influenza appear on this list.

Indecision and procrastination, the patterns of thinking that ready the body for viruses, occur throughout our lives. They do not always cause death nor do they always produce a cold or the flu. What they do cause is a susceptibility, a weakness, in the body that makes the virus' objective easier for it to accomplish. What is that microorganism's goal in life? To survive. It wants to share your body and does most of the time without you even knowing. But when the attitudes are conducive to an attack of influenza a war begins. Fighting the virus is what gives you the symptoms we commonly endure without benefit of cure. When a cold or flu gets the better of you, be assured somewhere in your life you have been indecisive, hesitating or procrastinating on courses of action that are productive.

To heal, determine where the indecision is, resolve the issue, follow through on your decision, and your body will immediately become stronger.

7)   Diabetes

As detailed in John Clark's story the mental construction creating diabetes is a refusal to give. It is often hard to see because most diabetics appear outwardly generous. They give frequently, but their giving always has a price tag. Ideas that "the world, the government, my father, you, owe me" are common in the way this person views life. When they give they expect something in return, otherwise they do not give. This deliberate withholding of self from others is characteristic of the thought patterns feeding pancreatic disorder. For John the accompanying attitude of "fear of never being able to have enough" manifested in excesses: indiscriminate eating, party binges, and other displays of irresponsibility. The fear becomes the impetus to take what you can when you can. John's thinking during his youth that he might as well do it all now, and later he'd deal with what might happen propelled him into a dangerous lifestyle that has indeed manifested his fears. Cultivating generosity, giving unconditionally, builds the thought pattern that enables this person to begin using their energies, particularly talents and skills, fruitfully.

8)   Suicide

The ultimate refusal to learn and cause change is to quit, "check out," "end it all," commit suicide.

On the surface it might seem that someone who commits suicide is someone who sees no alternatives in life and so chooses death. The truth is there are always alternatives, sometimes they are unpleasant, even repugnant, but they are alternatives nonetheless. Thus one who commits suicide is not a victim at all, unless it is of his or her own poor judgement. Rather they are stuck in denial that change needs to occur – most often a misdeed they do not want to face and correct, unwanted pregnancy, adultery, embezzlement. In rare instances suicide is a result of anger, a desire to hurt someone else, revenge. This most often occurs with adolescents. Most failed suicides are a result of bargaining. The thinking follows the lines of "maybe someone will find me before I die, if so my life will change." Many times those committing suicide are trapped in the depression of fighting change without ever coming to the point of acceptance. Killing the body is the only end they can see to their misery. For a person like these, acceptance only comes when they end physical life.

What they do not realize is the hardship this brings to their soul, for whatever was unresolved in the life still needs to be resolved when the body no longer exists. Death does not change the inner consciousness, it merely disconnects it from the bodily shell. Far from being left behind him, the essence of what the suicide was trying to escape remains with him.

To initiate a new pattern of thinking, accept that there is no escape from judgement. Ultimately, the only one who judges you, your soul growth, is you.

You are the only one who has to live with you, others choose you. There must be a reason, ask them what it is.

Come out of your self-pity by helping those less fortunate than yourself. Helping others has a wonderful way of putting your own life into perspective.

9)   *Human Immunodeficiency Virus (AIDS)*

It is not coincidence that the first identifiable cases of human immunodeficiency virus (HIV) which precedes the development of acquired immune deficiency syndrome was in male homosexuals. HIV is caused by defensiveness stemming from insecurity in the identity, how one sees self. Whether you believe homosexuality is right or wrong, a choice or a genetic condition, there is no denying that it has not been acceptable in our society. For the most part it has been behavior that has remained hidden from employers, landlords, friends, and as long as possible wives. Living a life of deceit produces an attitude that others are against you, even when they are not. This in turn feeds the defensiveness which becomes a vicious pattern that weakens mind and body. The attitude of feeling power-less is common in hemophiliacs, and often in those who require blood transfusions, who must deal with always being at risk of bleeding to death. The fact that the disease is highly and easily transmittable through sexual contact also brings these mental energy patterns into focus, for there are many who have been exposed but are immune.

As long as you believe the world is against you it is. For the way you construct your thinking defines the kind, quality, and reality of your life. As a man thinketh, so is he. To conquer this self-defeating pattern of thinking you will need to give up any attachment to being a target for others' negativity, a victim.

Cultivate open-mindedness. Be willing to believe the best about others, situations, life. Meditate so you can begin knowing yourself as a spiritual being, a child of the Source, the Creator. Identifying yourself beyond the physical is an important step toward claiming the power you possess. That power is the realization that thought is cause. Make sure yours are creating what you want.

10)   Homicide

It is not simplistic to say that murder only occurs where there is a lack of respect for life and a lack of self control. It is the root of the classical debate on-going in all societies concerning the death penalty for those who break the laws of trust that hold a society together and the aborting of fetuses that are dependent upon the female's body for survival. These issues polarize society for people will favor one and reject the other. Moreover they polarize individuals, the ultimate struggle for a reasoner is when good and evil are unresolved. This conflict epitomizes the construction of thinking that leads to taking another's life. Murder is in defiance of what is at least acceptable behavior and at most morally sound as reflected in the teachings of all great spiritual masters and a majority of manmade laws.

When man can take control of his capacity to learn, channeling it toward understanding himself and his fellow man, we can hope to see a transition here. Only as man releases himself from the animal nature of his body and aligns himself with the intuitive nature of his spirit will he rise above the dictates of the survival instinct. I believe this transformation in consciousness is happening even now as we progress into the 21st century.

In every case the thoughts that cause us harm can be changed. They will not be changed by lawsuits. They will not be changed by ignoring them or hoping they die out with a generation. They can be replaced by new ways of thinking. Ways that reflect understanding born from self-knowledge used for self-realization. History is filled with true stories of everyday heroes. People who inspire us to live better, treat each other better, be better.

Change will come as we learn to harmonize with the way of the universe, as we respect its rules of conduct, its governing laws. We will move beyond this present stage of evolution – one filled with the growing pains of leaving compulsiveness behind in favor of reasoning – as we uphold timeless principles of higher-mindedness and righteous conduct. The changes we make in ourselves will transform our world. By demonstrating greater love and concern for our fellow man, we will replace the negative patterns with ways of thinking that heal ourselves and each other. We will initiate the ways of Spiritual Man.

"*Caring parents produce healthier adults.*"

That was a front page headline in *USA Today* [March 7, 1996], a national newspaper in the United States. It caught my attention because I wondered who was not aware of this truth that they would feel the need to scientifically verify it. The accompanying story explained that a 35-year study following 87 Harvard College men into middle age reported that the healthiest at age 55 were those who at age 20 reported that their parents were most caring. Young men who said their parents were less loving, especially those who saw their parents as unjust, were most apt to have illnesses like heart disease and hypertension by 55.

This research supports what many people believe: that what we think and how we feel about *each other* determines our ease or dis-ease. Your fiancee makes your heart race while your boss is a pain in the neck. For me, as a metaphysician, this study verifies a more advanced concept of wholistic health: the undeniable health effects of *mental* heredity. Most mainstream researchers won't go near this idea because of the current wave of victims that permeates our global society. The way you think directly affects the condition of your body? No, that can't be! Well, maybe as far as those thoughts that allow you to smoke ever-increasing numbers of cigarettes or the ones that tell you it's okay to eat dessert today because you'll exercise tomorrow. Now *those* thoughts can affect your health.

And maybe as this study suggests, *"the perception of being loved may lower stress hormones and improve immune function."* So maybe the more we love and are loved, the healthier we can expect to be. But can we really believe that the way we *think* contributes to illness? Sure, we have all known someone who had a will to live, a drive to recover. And they did. They threw off the shackles of disease and reorganized their thinking and their lives, and to this day tell the story.

Can we go so far as to hypothesize that the way someone *thinks* can make him have a heart attack? We've all heard of someone who died of a broken heart. Perhaps it's more than a metaphor. Perhaps it is symbolic to describe the causal thought of a breakdown in the physical body.

But dare we conclude that the way someone thinks causes him to be a diabetic? Surely not. To have cancer? No way, say those entrenched in allopathic medicine, and denial. After all, that would be blaming the victim of the disease, the person who is already suffering enough.

Yet what is it that makes one person welcome death, closing his lifetime in peaceful dignity, while another rails angrily, poisoning his final days by refusing to surrender to the inevitable? What motivates one person to greatness from a misfortune, while another crumples never recovering from a tragedy?

It is universally true that the quality of our thinking determines the quality of the lives we lead. This is true whether we speak of our friends, our chosen careers, our health. When we think positively and with love, we find the magic in life. We receive good fortune. We expect miracles and we witness them.

The ways of the universe are a mystery only to those who refuse to see the truth that eternally applies to us all. "As above, so below". "As a man thinketh, so is he." As a metaphysician, I would describe it as thought is cause and the physical is its manifest likeness.

Man can be a victim of his own limited thinking. He can fill his mind with fear and hatred, and his body with imbalance and disease. Man can also transcend any limitation. He can learn from hardship. He need not become helpless, bitter, or self-pitying. He can draw upon strengths he did not know he had. Certainly Helen Keller spoke with authority when she warned, *"Self pity is our worst enemy and if we yield to it we can never do anything wise in the world."*

At this stage of humanity's development, the consciousness of our world is continually being drawn toward health. Too often the importance of health and the ways to achieve it are lost amid the fearful warnings of well-intentioned leaders and professionals. Approaching health from the standpoint of illness and disease is like putting a cart before the horse for as American philosopher Ralph Waldo Emerson noted over a century ago, *"sickness is poor-spirited."* There might be times when the extreme measures of modern science are required to eradicate the effects of inharmonies in mind and body, yet who wants to live a life fearing disease and dreading physical debilitation? Such a person is poor-spirited and his life is laid waste by the poverty of ignorance. There are better ways to think, and better ways to live.

Emerson was not a stranger to Universal Truth. He knew the origin of mankind's health lies in the purity of his thinking. His acquaintance with transcendent wisdom shines in his writings: *"The first wealth is health. Sickness is poor-spirited, and cannot serve any one; it must husband its resources to live. But health answers its own ends, and has to spare; runs over, and inundates the neighborhoods and creeks of other men's necessities."* Emerson knew health is necessary for spiritual generosity between people.

Therein lies the secret in the revelation that "caring parents produce healthier adults." Researchers stressed that the type of parents you had or the type of parent you are to your children determines health decades into the future. Love and wisdom from our first teachers, our parents, lay an incomparable foundation for every child. The more obscure truth revealed in this study is found not in what it says about what is received but rather what it says about giving. This study beautifully illustrates that parents who care, who actively love, are healthier *from* and *because of* the loving. The universal command to love others as you love yourself can now take on greater meaning for it is a cornerstone for health.

Every culture in the world encourages a richness of spirit. Each teaches a principle of how to establish healthy human relations, how to get along with one another. This concept is described in every holy scripture because it is the original cause for compassion, cooperation, and goodwill among people. Too often the truth eludes us because we react to the way that truth is expressed.

Older scriptures describe this principle in a negative form: *"Hurt not others in ways that you yourself would find hurtful"* (Udana-Varga of Buddhism), *"What is hateful to you, do not do to your fellow man. That is the entire Law; all the rest is commentary."* (Talmud of Judaism), or *"This is the sum of duty: do naught unto others which would cause you pain if done to you"* (Mahabarata of Hinduism).

The more recently written scriptures, the Christian Bible's *"Love ye one another"* and the Islamic Koran's *"No one of you is a believer until he desires for his brother that which he desires for himself,"* tell us how to fulfill the law.

Self Revelation
When an Analysis Spans a Lifetime

I had heard thousands of analyses, personally transcribed several hundred, and I had never encountered one that opened like this:

> *We see there is an attachment to a male form.*

Unconsciously verifying the truth of the intuitive insight, immediately I was besieged by emotion; surprise, fear, rejection, embarrassment, hurt. I had received one other Intuitive Health Analysis two years before, and I could tell in these ten words that this one was going to far surpass it in what it revealed about me.

I was not disappointed.

This analysis went far beyond my immediate health condition. It brought significant lifetime issues to the forefront of my thinking. In so doing it addressed karmic issues of perfection and authority that I had been aware of and struggled with since adolescence. What I did not realize until this analysis was how I tied these unfulfilled desires, these misconceptions and problems, to the "male form" in my life.

Using this analysis, attending to its insight and heeding its advice, would prove to be one of the most powerful tools for change in my life. In so many ways this Intuitive Health Analysis is spanning an entire lifetime.

I was present when this analysis was conducted. Upon hearing the opening line, I first thought the male it spoke of was the man in my life, my significant other in common vernacular. I was constantly dealing with emotional struggles concerning our private life, which in retrospect existed in my imagination. He had been married for years even before I was born and had five grown children, and he was not inclined toward commitment during this latter part of his life. So I found myself, a 22-year-old who believed in fairy tales, committed to a man who fancied himself a modern Cassanova, making up for lost time and seeking revenge on all females for imagined hurt his wife had inflicted upon him. Eventually those attitudes produced his early and ugly demise. The Cassanova part I knew about, the vengeance I would soon come to know.

Unlike many women, I did not entertain ideas of changing him as a potential mate. I knew that was not possible. I did believe my loving him could have a positive influence. I believed our ideals were similar, though I admitted that our practice of those ideals differed greatly. And that bothered me. Years later I would realize that was a key to the lesson I needed to learn that was revealed in this analysis. But at the time I received this information, I had yet to acquire the wisdom that is coming to me even now. Then, I was constantly asking myself, "why do you stay with this man?" Although I loved the innovative parts of his thinking, I was finding some of his actions questionable and therefore was beginning to question my association with him. That was why when the analysis opened with "attachment to a male form" I thought of him.

At the time of the analysis, I was 26 and he was twice my age, and all the myths and tales of the May-December romances applied even though part of me denied them for years. The younger one's desire for the sagacity revealed with age, the older's yearning for the freshness of youth. In all honesty, there were ego perks on both sides. He didn't offer me physical wealth or fame, he afforded me the benefit of experience. His thinking was extensive and visionary, focused on things in and beyond the physical world, surpassing that of anyone else I had met. I more than learned from him. In the beginning I drew etheric sustenance from his ideas to fuel my own inner drive and passion to understand the meaning of life. Fresh out of college and wanting to somehow make the world a better place, I was a most eager and willing student.

It was this mental attraction that drew us together. Initially we seemed mentally compatible in mutually beneficial ways. Attachment was an appropriate word to describe my thoughts toward this man. I believed it was this mental attachment more than an emotional one that sustained our relationship for fifteen years. Yet this was a difficult area for me to be honest with myself as the analysis noted:

> ....We see the emotions relating to that of the mental in as much as the intensity that has been given is reflected in the emotions. This emotional tendency then would create the attachment toward people but we see this one does not allow herself to maintain this consciously. We see that it is a way of punishing the self for we see the desire is to associate with people closely, but we see the fear involved also that if the associations were close this one would be hurt in some way or the other. We do see this as loosening over a period of time, but we do see more conscious attention needed in this area. We do see there is a great desire to be honest with the self but we do see times of her deviating from this because she becomes attached to fulfillment of a certain area and forgets another at these times...

As time went by it became increasingly clear that as long as I remained the student to his teacher the association was endearing and rewarding. As the years passed, the security I gleaned from my learning and experience led to conflicts between us.

It would be years before I would come to realize there never was a future with this man. My desire to live a fairy tale would never find fruition with him, and for very good reasons. The downfall of this association was due to the classic reasons that such archetypal relationships disappear – a lack of common goals and interests. We were not together for romance, we were together for education. The more I grew in my teaching the less he grew in his.

My failure was being blinded by the attachment I knew existed and, when I was willing to clearly perceive, being too afraid of his wrath to change. I had put the teacher on a pedestal when I first met him, endowing him with virtues he did not possess and dismissing the weaknesses he did. I pretended he was something he was not. I would be able to admit the truth of my attachment only after he had been dead for some time and I no longer feared repercussions. The way his life ended, a decade after this reading, stimulated more awarenesses. Having admitted my failures, I could see his was failing to meet the potential he saw, he pretended to be something he was not. He did not practice what he preached, and all the while hated himself for it; this eventually brought his death from lung cancer.

The story about this man is relevant not only because he was the first person that came to mind when I heard my analysis but because, as my awarenesses unfolded, I realized he was representative of another man in my life. A man who not coincidentally also died of cancer in 1990, just three weeks before the teacher. My grandfather.

I struggled a while with who the analysis was referencing – my teacher or my grandfather. The answer was in the analysis all the time:

> *We see there is an attachment to a male form. We see this to be in the past and we see this one has allowed this to color the thinking at the present time.*

"We see this to be in the past."   When I finally let those words sink in I realized this part of the analysis could not be talking about the teacher. It was talking about someone who had been in my life a much longer time.

My grandfather, who was still living when I received the analysis, was physically much more a part of my past than my present. He lived in a small Missouri town while I lived hundreds of miles away in New Orleans. When it dawned on me that *he* was the *"male form"* the accompanying awarenesses were overwhelming. Without a doubt I carried my grandfather with me every day of my life. I don't know when, or if, I would have realized how much so without the benefit of this analysis. This intuitive insight into my thinking has been a godsend for me for years. I knew my grandfather blessed me at times, plagued me at others, but until the analysis I had yet to admit just how much of my thinking was entwined in who he was and his profound influence on my early life that had set the patterns I lived by.

Once I was willing to admit it, the truth was so obvious. In fact it's an excellent example of how my *"attachment to a male form"* could blind my vision, keeping me from seeing the obvious. The evening this analysis was done, I had driven two hundred miles from a visit with my family. I had left following a heated contest of egos with my grandfather, a too common occurrence since before I left home for college. It seemed like every visit was punctuated with a verbal tennis match. Our bone of contention was religion, and neither of us ever won although every time he bested me in rhetoric. Throughout the duration of the drive I had been thinking and reacting, thinking and reacting, trying to sort out why our discussions always seemed to turn out the same way, why I let him manipulate me emotionally, why I couldn't keep my mouth shut and when I couldn't why he wasn't willing to listen or give me the benefit of the doubt. This was what I was allowing *"to color the thinking at the present time"*.

> *We see there is a need to refer back into that past experience and to understand it more fully so that this one may release this individual with understanding. We see this as having produced within this one a sense of competition.*

Once I knew I was encountering my grandfather, I experienced a freedom. I wanted to understand our relationship, good and bad, and I was not afraid, as I was with the teacher, to face whatever might come to me.

In specific ways we were very much alike, my grandfather and I. Part of this was his influence in raising me which was considerable since we lived in the same household until I was twelve. The other part was the similar lacks we shared in our understandings. We were both willful and stubborn, persuasive and domineering, empathetic and overly sensitive, altruistic and self-centered. The way we interacted had certainly produced a sense of competition in me. It had positively fueled a passion within me to help others, as I had seen him do so often. He was generous and kind. When he gave, he gave in a big way. It never appeared that he expected anything in return from most people, although I had long known the closer you were to him the more he demanded. Negatively the competition fueled a passion within me to be understood. When I was young this centered more on agreement, the type I witnessed in my grandfather. His whole life was built around swaying people to his way of thinking. He felt it was his calling to bring people to God. In my 20's I often felt my calling was to bring them to personal accountability. Much later I would realize these passions were described in my analysis:

...We do see a strong drive within this one. We see there is difficulty at times to use the gentleness of self and reflecting into this motivating force for we see that this one has met many desires and wants for self. We see that this produces a state of intensity for herself. We see it is very difficult to express energy as a result of this intensity. We see that she will become blocked easily in the expression for we see it is pressing from within herself outward in the attempts to express outwardly, consciously...

The problems between us were accentuated because his ministry diminished, the equivalent for him of ceasing to learn, from the time I was born. At the time of the analysis, I was finding my own way in life, my ministry was just beginning and it was not the same as his. I know that was a disappointment to him because he had offered to pay to put me through school at a Christian college (I went to the University of Missouri on a Curator's scholarship). I also know my choosing my own path in life in some ways was a failure in his eyes of his ability to persuade.

Although my choice for learning was not made with him in mind, it was not a personal affront to him, it probably appeared so because our discussions could so easily turn into arguments where someone had to be right and someone had to be wrong. The competition manifested as "my way is better than your way." It was a constant source of pain to me because each time I wanted him to understand me, and when he didn't I tried to make him understand. Each time I failed. The analysis told me why in the opening paragraph:

We see there is an intense quality as relating to the need to succeed that is reflective of this individual, this past association, and we see that this causes this one at times to lose the focus of attention on those situations that would be most helpful in producing learning for herself.

For months I studied this analysis. First it dawned in my consciousness that this analysis was talking about a relationship that had been with me far beyond the four year duration with the teacher. Second, I realized its applications in regard to my relationship with my grandfather. Third, I began seeing the similarities between these two men in my life and identifying my common reactions to them. This was amazing to me. I had studied the psychological ideas of how women marry their fathers, and somewhere down the line I admitted these associations fell into that category.

However, within two years of receiving this analysis I was certified as a psiologist, what can briefly be described as an intuitively-skilled counselor. Part of my training was resolving this personal issue. To my learned way of thinking the repetition signified karmic lessons yet to be learned. It was like I hadn't quite made the grade in the "grandfather class" in this earthly schoolroom so I was in the "teacher class" still trying to pass the course. Thanks to the spiritual disciplines – particularly meditation – that I practiced daily plus the intuitively-based self-counseling, I was able to make great progress. I began to see that beyond having similar men in my life I was repeating *patterns of thinking* in my interaction with men like these. Patterns that affected my ability to think clearly, patterns that were wearing on my health.

As I moved farther away from focusing on interactions with these two men I was free to delve into my consciousness, not what I thought about them but what I thought about *me*. First, I worked on changing my thoughts which were aptly described in my analysis. This prepared me for the next level of awareness. Just when I would get to the point of thinking I had gleaned all I could from the information I received, a new insight would surface. It was exhilarating and exhausting, this process of releasing attachment.

It was also important to my physical health. Except for yearly colds that when younger included bronchitis, and occasional tension headaches now, I was very healthy. The analysis verified this, citing areas affected by the detrimental patterns of thinking:

> *...We see the physical body somewhat rigid at this point. We see that this is again reflected by this great drive and motivation to express self. We see that as a result there is tension created in all parts of the body.... (it is) not allowed to function at its full capacity.*

The reading covered where I knew I had some difficulty. It was clear that my thoughts and emotions affected my body. *"The systems of release are not functioning at full rate"* which produced disturbances in *"the lung tissue, the skin, easily overloaded digestive system"*. My headaches were the result of muscular *"tightness on either side of the cervical region...producing a pressure sensation at the cerebellum and lower occipital lobe. We see (because of) this posture.. the body becomes worn and tired and the toxins do not leave this area, thus we see this would produce a pressure sensation or a type of headache at this point.* This also explained how and why I experienced repeated fatigue that often interfered with my ability to focus my attention and think clearly.

The analysis covered several other issues, from impatience to communication. It offered suggestions on how to consistently cause what I wanted and how to incorporate more people into my life. As I responded to the considerable information I had received, I found my body to be a gauge letting me know when I was making true progress and when I might be getting off track. Wholistic health was taking on greater meaning every day.

Significant advances were made in liberating my consciousness when I could finally see how this analysis was addressing issues that transcended my physical life. These were issues that touched my soul. Lessons in life, understandings from experience, that my soul needed to learn in order to be whole and complete. That is why this analysis was given to me when it was. A cosmic gift of intuitive awareness just out of my grasp at the time, and exactly what I needed to propel my awareness forward for the next twenty years.

Ultimately what this analysis stimulated in me was Self realization of the most sublime. Both men afforded me a place to learn and deepen understandings that would be added to my soul. They afforded me the opportunity to give without attachment, without conditions. Because of who they were they stimulated in me a necessary ego transformation, a change that would free me to give without obligating the receiver.

In my early life I wanted to give back to my grandfather even a part of what he had given me. I knew what he wanted most from me was for me to follow in his footsteps which I could not in good conscience do. So I never felt what I gave him was good enough, and often what I did give was rejected. In time I admitted *I* was the one who decided that there was something wrong with me because I couldn't give him what he wanted. If I had understood this, I would have been at peace with myself, regardless of what he thought. It would be years before I would be a peace. Later it was my teacher with whom I felt this overpowering urge to give. Again I was trying to repay someone for what they had given me. This time I did try to give what I felt was wanted from me, again doubting that what I offered was good enough and often feeling rejected. My problem was insecurity in the value of what I had to offer, so at times I would petulantly argue with grandfather, rebelling, and at times with the teacher I would feign indifference. I believed what I wanted to give, what I had to offer was worthwhile, honest, and loving but I was never quite sure and I looked to them for the knowing I did not know how to give to myself. In both cases validation was only forthcoming when it would aggrandize the men, pay them in ways they expected.

Eventually I realized I was wrong. I had no right to take from these men what they did not want to, or could not, give. Particularly when what I wanted could only be self-produced. The security, the trust, I was lacking would only come from my own efforts, my capacity to transform belief into knowing.

....We do see that there are doubts as to what she has to offer to other people. We see this is the conscious mind placing limits upon herself. We do see there is a need for this one to simply trust – to trust in the conscious and subconscious harmonization in pulling out that which is needed in each individual situation...

Eventually I saw the doubts caused me to question my own motives needlessly, and to my own harm. Yes, others could believe in me, could even know what I could do, but until I made the transformation no amount of influence would make the truth real to me. This meant I had to change my ego, my sense of who I was. I saw it as maturing, growing up. It was a challenge. I wanted to be honest, for I valued Universal Truth above all things, in fact I had set my greatest desire to be able to think and act in alignment at all times. Striving to accomplish this desire was the catalyst that gave me the vehicle for change.

As I learned this lesson the next level of it became apparent. Once I was secure in what I offered, I still faced attachments. Now I could finally see my problem, a truer attachment, was I wanted these men to *receive* what I offered. I wanted acknowledgement, not validation, of the gift. I wanted them to understand, to respect me and my efforts, even when they did not agree. When this was not forthcoming as I imagined I was hurt, or rejected, or angry, or embarrassed. My attachment never was to these men in my life.

After all this time, all the insights gained, all the lessons learned, what I uncovered as the cause of my distress was simple, concise, piercing. The attachment was to "the male form", the image of the act of giving I had made. That image was the male form, not the men in my life. I had created a thinking pattern of self-doubt that was stimulated anytime I wanted someone to receive what I had to give. Which was often, since I was teaching, lecturing, counseling, doing talk radio, and constantly in the public eye. As I expanded my consciousness to realize the impact of "the attachment to a male form" I found all aspects of my life, every relationship with others transformed.

All along I was restless. I was growing but the growth sometimes damaged my mind and body. I had learned that change did not have to be painful, in fact I knew the kind of transformation that feeds the soul is not a cause for harm. It doesn't wound or make you heart-sick, it heals. When the soul learns it knows peace. My peace arrived in ever-deepening degrees paralleled by understanding that male form.

The attachment existed as long as I needed to learn how to give openly and freely. Learn I did in so many experiences spanning forty years. When speaking of how I would form *"close and meaningful associations that produce much sharing"* my analysis had said the changes I needed to make *"will be alleviated only by the consistent and conscious effort to change this mind pattern."* This was true in my associations with hundreds of people through those years. Teachers, students, administrators, lawyers, doctors, young and old, rich and poor, American or European or African or Asian or Australian. My chosen life path brought to me people of all sizes, shapes, colors, a wealth of experiences for me to learn what this analysis so succinctly discerned.

I knew all along I had to do the work. This is why I made time daily for spiritual communion, mental disciplines, consciousness honing exercises. It was why I actively remembered and interpreted my dreams. It was why I devoted the majority of my time in service to others. I knew how to work to produce something worthwhile. I knew my work would eventually pay in the freedom I fervently desired. It did, but in a way I could not have anticipated in 1978.

For two decades I cherished unconditional love as an ideal worthy of pursuit. One I believed would be the cornerstone of peace of mind. Lessons in the earthly schoolroom showed me the limits of *pursuit,* the offspring of ego's motivation. And they opened my eyes to the expansiveness of *becoming,* the progeny of Self revelation. Even now, my husband will point out how I become obsessive, particularly when I grab every available moment to work at my computer on a treasured project at hand. Or how I will keep reiterating a point, keep after something, until it bears fruit. It is "the attachment to the male form" of my ideas. The creative fervor that arises within me cannot be denied. It can only be channeled, and it still generates that intensity that the analysis described so many years ago.

I have learned to respect that most powerful of energies – the Kundalini – for when I do I am richly rewarded and when I fail I know it immediately. I don't run from her anymore. I no longer try to escape her through alcohol, or drugs, or sleep. I court her more consistently, no longer a favorite during creative periods and an outcast during dry periods. Now I wrestle with divine beings more often than demons. Both are a challenge but I'll choose the divine every time.

Above all, I have learned that *being* is the state of consciousness that enriches my soul. Attachment dissipates, creation flourishes in the reality of being. For me it is the loving union of freedom and responsibility, the marriage made in Heaven and consummated in how I live my life.

*E*very time I study this analysis, done for me two decades ago, I learn something new about myself. Even though I have committed its words to memory, the insights continue to come to me with each review. No matter how many analyses I read, I am continually amazed at what they can offer.

For me, this analysis spans my lifetime. It reveals karmic indentures and genetic mind patterns that I meet again and again in my life as I endeavor to climb the evolutionary ladder toward Enlightenment. It describes them clearly and concisely, helping me to focus on the learning that I am here to do. To, in the truest sense of the word, make myself whole. And when I think about how profound that is – to know why you are here – I am filled with gratitude that this means of Self awareness is in the world today.

The Quest for Permanent Healing

Awareness is a giant step toward realization, just as desire is the major component to attainment.

An Intuitive Health Analysis reveals the metaphysical and physical transformations that will ensure wholeness and health. Most people readily respond to the suggestions for the physical body. They procure the vitamins or herbs, adjust diet, seek the suggested health practitioners. These do give symptomatic relief. This is the movement from awareness to realization.

How readily people respond to the mental and emotional parts of the analysis depends upon their readiness for change. Some are ready to take greater control of the life, some are relieved to discover "why", some are tired of fighting. The depth of the analysis' insights are guided by the individual's willingness to become *self*-aware. This is a challenge for anyone. It is a challenge to be met by the serious aspirant, the courageous, the one who is prepared to enter a new realm of self-discovery. Intuitive Health Analyses fully used, elevate your awareness thereby lifting you to your next cycle of growth.

Responding to suggestions for mental and emotional change also depends upon the individual's desire for permanent healing for it is eliminating the disorder where it begins that cures. Freeing our spirits of the demons that sometimes take up residence in the corners of our minds need not be frightening or even arduous work. In fact the mental condition necessary for spiritual healing to arise is actually one where hope and love have replaced fear and doubt.

The role of spirit in healing is witnessed every day, in every culture. The word *spirit* comes from the Latin *spiritus* meaning *breath*. Spirit is breath, life, vitality, vital spirit, soul, consciousness, psyche. It is the attitude, thought, idea, inspiration, feeling, inclination, impulse. Man has created all manner of mechanical devices to maintain the physical body, to keep it nourished, to keep it breathing. But when the spirit of the person is absent, only the shell remains and when artificial life support systems are removed, the soul is finally free to continue its journey. The inseparable link between the state of one's soul and the state of one's body is a testimony to the Universal Truth *thought is cause and the physical is its manifest likeness.* The connection between spirit and body has been professed religiously for millennia and debated in scientific circles for fifteen hundred years. Religion seeks to live that Truth, and science seeks to define It. Their quests lead to the same destination although few today recognize that truth.

Universal Truths are illustrated in the parables and allegories of every Holy Scripture of the world. From the *Koran* of the Muslim to the *I Ching* of Confucianism, from the Jewish *Talmud* to Native American Indian prayers and lore, all cultures have a philosophy that ministers to the spirit, guiding thinking toward wholeness. *Thought is cause* is one of these Truths that are universal, applying to anyone, any time, anywhere.

When the Jew or the Christian speaks of "purifying his temple" he is not talking about vacuuming his church. He means praying to cleanse his mind and fasting to cleanse his physical body, the temple of his soul. The Hebrew prophet Isaiah wrote, *"Wash yourselves, make yourselves clean; remove the evil of your doings from before my eyes. Cease to do evil, learn to do good. Seek justice, correct oppression."* The evil of your doings is any ill intent behind your actions. Thought is cause. Know your intentions, know your thoughts. Make them good, productive, helpful, cooperative, is the message for and about the spirit.

Accounts of the teaching and ministry of Jesus of Nazareth, in the New Testament of the Bible include many miraculous healings. Before he healed the sick he would ask his patient, *"Do you believe?"* Jesus understood the power of thought and he harmonized with the Universal Laws. An assertion of faith upon the part of the sick is necessary for healing to be permanent, *thought is cause.*

Awareness is the first step toward realization. It was true two thousand years ago, it is still true today.

The Hindu's challenge for wholeness appears in the form of the three principles of nature which manifest themselves in every person, the three great gunas: Sattvas or truth, Rajas or passion, and Tamas or indifference.

The Hindu believe that when wisdom is present, Sattvas is the ruling guna. *Thought is cause*, and wisdom frees man from all manners of blindness and limitation. The Laws of Manu say, *"The body is cleansed by water, the internal organ is purified by truthfulness, the individual soul by sacred learning and austerities, the intellect by true knowledge."*

For the Buddhist wholeness is personified as Buddhic consciousness, the illumined state of awareness. One who aspires to become enlightened comes to realize it is the action of the mind that determines the state of one's consciousness. *Thought is cause.*

> *"It is like a painter*
> *Spreading the various colors:..*
> *That mind never stops,*
> *Manifesting all forms,*
> *countless, inconceivably many,*
> *unknown to one another...*
> *Mind is like an artist,*
> *Able to paint the world:..*
> *If people know the actions of mind*
> *Create all the worlds,*
> *They will see the Buddha*
> *And understand Buddha's true nature...*
> *If people want to really know*
> *All Buddhas of all times,*
> *They should contemplate the nature of the cosmos:*
> *All is but mental construction."* – Garland Sutra 20

The Universal Laws are described in every Holy Scripture on Earth. Truth is what makes them endure, generation after generation. Regardless of the generation's virtue or vice, the Truth endures and so man's descriptions of that Truth are ageless. Writings and oral stories embodying these truths are healing. They enrich the spirit, mind, and body.

Whether parable, myth, or allegory they are penned in symbols that strike the universal chord. They speak to everyone living now. They speak to those who lived five thousand years ago, and to those who will live five thousand years hence. Like family genealogies tracing physical roots, these holy works when studied in the language of the soul, which SOM researchers have named the Universal Language of Mind, reveal the origin and evolution of mankind and all creation in our universe. They tell us where we have come from. And they tell us where we are going.

For this reason every religion encourages Self awareness. Each delineates the path to enlightenment. The tendency for separation and division, a result of losing sight of the quest to manifest spiritual ideals, feeds religion's descent into dogma. "My God is the only true God." "Everyone must be converted, be saved, believe as we do." "They are not like us and therefore are evil, are to be shunned, are destined to destruction, are appointed to die." "There is nothing you can do to alter our lot in life." The statements may sound extreme but they are the simple roots of what is harmful in man's practice of religion. Such statements and the enmity they produce are a reflection of man's own thinking, the limits of the ego of the masses. Within the individual they are the seed of disease.

Consensus does not create Truth. Agreement does not produce Truth. Soon we will realize this. Soon we will admit that Truth exists independent of man's reason. The best part of religion is its capacity to summon the cornerstone of man's imaginative power – faith. Faith in something greater than ourselves. Faith in what is good, what is right. Faith in a power beyond our own. Half of hospitalized male patients indicate religion helps them cope with their illness, one in five say religion is "the most important thing that keeps me going."

Studies substantiate the healing impact of faith. Those who practice their religion have one half the risk of heart attack and lower blood pressure even after controlling for the effects of smoking and socioeconomic status. Patients undergoing open-heart surgery who practice a religion are three times more likely to survive than those who have none. Religious beliefs counteract feelings of helplessness, providing meaning and order to challenging life situations and restoring a sense of control. *Thought is cause.* Cultivating rich religious beliefs, pursuing Truth that is universal, improves mental and physical health as well as spiritual well-being.

The capacity to believe Truth is only the beginning of awareness, not the end. Soon we will release the chains of prejudice, freeing our minds and hearts to live the teachings of the greatest masters who ever walked on this planet. We will realize believing is the mental preparation that gives us conscience while motivating us toward knowing the Truth. Living it. Becoming it.

Every religion teaches the Truth of how to get along with your neighbor. Most state it in the negative form, "do no harm...", yet the idea of what to do is borne from the restraint of what not to do. We will see more insight and instruction in what to do in the coming centuries. As we mature beyond reasoning into developing intuition we will find wholeness in Self and among ourselves. Living peacefully begins by thinking peacefully. *Thought is cause.* We will love one another and by the loving realize the path to enlightenment is one path traveled by many.

The Truth is every religion teaches Self discipline, for from discipline comes Self control which leads to mastery. The great masters throughout our history have known this. It is how they lived and what they taught. Their teachings are universally true and that is why religions were borne from their teaching. The Truth is mastery is every man's destiny.

In the 21st century we will witness a new respect for those who have traveled the path before us, and we will recognize there are those among us who are both farther along the path than ourselves and those who have yet to reach the heights we have attained.

This awareness, a significant destination on the path to enlightenment, is found where philosophy and conduct intersect, where religion and science unite, where thought is cause and the physical is its manifest likeness.

F or the past 1500 years, man has been pursuing a contemplation he calls science.

Although it has often seemed at odds with religion, science nevertheless owes its innovativeness and progress to man's capacity to dream, to imagine, to *think*. The thinkers among us, apart from their paths in physical life, are the ones who display the genius needed to lead mankind. Unlike those who support the status quo, they are constantly moving beyond the perimeters of what already exists. While others prescribe drugs that do not eliminate disease or change ageless messages of truth to suit the tastes of today, these men and women seek *cures* to the ills of mankind. These people seek the Truth about health and healing.

And so at the dawn of the next thousand years, we find *thought is cause* appearing in more scientific journals than most status quo physicians realize. These visionary physicians have seen evidence of the power of thought to heal. Rather than ignore it or leave it to someone else, they are determined to prove the connection between faith and healing. They believe the answers will enable them to be better physicians to those in need. For instance, a 1988 study by Dr. Randolph Byrd of 393 patients at the San Francisco General Hospital coronary-care unit found those who were prayed for had fewer cases of congestive heart failure, less pneumonia, less need for antibiotics and fewer cardiac arrests than those who weren't. A 1995 study at the Dartmouth Medical School of 232 patients who had undergone elective heart surgery found the "very" religious were three times more likely to recover than those who were not.

Of 300 studies on spirituality in scientific journals, the National Institute for Healthcare Research found nearly three-fourths showed that religion had a positive effect on health. "Research also shows four out of five patients want doctors to ask them about their faith, and one in two want their doctors to pray with them," says the Institute's president, David Larson. Yet only an estimated 10% of patients say their doctors talk to them about their faith as a factor in their healing.

The common consensus among scientists is that doctors who recognize the advantage of faith in recovery cannot instruct patients without faith to get it. There is no drug that can supply it. Scientists do not believe that patients who learn of the relationship of faith to recovery can suddenly develop the faith that they do not have. Even if most have not witnessed, and definitely haven't experienced, the kind of quantum change man is capable of, at least science is moving in the direction that will eventually lead to this "discovery." As C. Everett Koop, former U.S. Surgeon General, describes this truth is revealed through experience, "Having, for many years, dealt with people of faith in regard to their own illnesses and those of their children, I have come to understand some things. People of faith have a different world view from those who do not have faith. They believe in the sovereignty of a God who makes no mistakes, and they believe as Robert Browning expressed it - 'Our times are in his hands who saith a whole, I planned; trust God see all, nor be afraid.' It seems that connection like this is good for the body, as well as the soul."

The reluctance with which such compliments are tendered reveals the enmity existing between the science of medicine and the philosophy of religion. Modern scientists and physicians have often been uncomfortable in the realm of faith. Yet with the undeniable connection between faith and healing, mind and body, both find themselves in this new milieu, seeking explanations in the scientific order already known to them. This is the heart of the School of Metaphysics' research, going beyond the limits previously accepted to understand the wholistic nature of man and his relationship to his universe. Faith becomes a needed precursor to knowing.

More and more scientists are admitting that spiritual beliefs form a vital part of the way we view life and death. They shape the way we think and determine the condition of our hearts in a literal sense as well as figurative. These beliefs are the impetus, the cause, for how we live them, the religion of our lives. They give us some very important necessities in life:

§ *A sense of meaning and purpose*

§ *A framework to set priorities and place stresses in perspective*

§ *Comfort in the face of illness and crisis*

§ *Support for a healthy lifestyle and avoidance of cigarettes, drugs, and alcohol*

§ *Opportunities for social contact and to develop supportive relationships*

§ *Reasons to be of service and help others*

§ *Sense of being part of something larger and feeling connected to something outside of oneself*

Religion at its highest manifestation is a wholistic philosophy of creation that pervades the consciousness and thus directs the life.

Science at its highest manifestation is an understanding of the cause and effect of creation that accelerates mankind's soul progression.

By uniting the two we discover our past and our future. When man believes with the intention to know, he realizes the power of his mind. He is free to use reasoning and intuition thus multiplying his understanding.

Intuition enables man to grasp the whole picture, reasoning gives him the ability to interpret the elements comprising the picture. For health and well-being he must be able to do both.

Because we stand on the threshold of the next evolutionary step, most of us are only now becoming more attentive to intuition in our lives. We have brief encounters with intuition that seem to come and go of their own bidding. Like children who haphazardly say a sound that meets with enthusiastic approval, we are just starting to use our minds intuitively, by accident. It was coincidence we say.

Intuitive Health Analyses elevate intuition above the level of chance. They represent years of study dedicated to understanding intuitive power, making it useful as a tool for health. Gratefully, they help us synthesize man's fourfold being: spiritual, mental, emotional, and physical. With intuition we can see the whole picture, the connections of the elements. Like the child who is learning to put words together to express his thoughts, we are just beginning to realize our potential. For such a person, the Intuitive Health Analysis becomes a series of lessons in four dimensions.

Faculty and researchers at the School of Metaphysics seek to transcend any discord between religion and science, uniting their quests. The course of study cultivates potential through progressive, daily disciplines which focus the mind and relax the body. By exercising reasoning and intuition, students release prejudices that limit their creativity and begin to freely use the Universal Laws that govern creation, the laws described in the holy text of every religion known to man. The world then becomes the student's laboratory; the place where his hypotheses are put to the test and new awarenesses are born. As the individual's consciousness becomes enlightened a new phase of growth is initiated, one we describe as Spiritual, Intuitive Man. This unifying of the mind and body frees the spirit, accelerating individual and collective evolution.

The Creator's Prodigy

The future is where ideas meet reality. When the dreams of today become the life we live. Where imagination realizes its power and memory knows its wisdom.

Our individual futures are the product of how often and how well we employ reasoning to guide our choices. Each individual chooses the people we will associate with, the songs we sing, the food we eat, the books we read, the thoughts that fill our minds. Each individual has every opportunity for growth and awareness, happiness and health, if he will only choose wisely. And as Jonas Salk remarked, "Wisdom is the fitness of the future." As individual sagacity increases, humanity's evolution will quicken.

It is mankind's destiny to be whole. And it is mankind's challenge to unite what seems dispersed, to join what seems separate. Mankind has two very strong forces pulling for it; the older is theology, the younger is science. Only through merging these two will mankind come into his own, meeting his challenge and realizing his destiny.

There are global patterns that reflect where we are collectively as a species. By drawing upon recently gleaned information, we can identify the probabilities into the third millennium for these patterns are far more than a listing of physical conditions. For instance in the World Health Organization's annual [1996] survey of the world's health, it was estimated that two billion people – 40% of the world's population – are sick at any given time. Comparative figures show this is a positive indication of improving health conditions because the percentage is shrinking. Overall, mankind is becoming healthier, primarily as a result of technology and education. Globally, the physical disorders leading to death are heart disease, pneumonia, and diarrhea, and poverty is cited as the biggest underlying cause. Poor living standards and conditions are a breeding ground for communicable disease.

Life expectancy varies widely. A person born in Uganda in 1993 will be lucky to survive to the mid-40's; a Japanese baby can expect to live to age 79. The USA, at a 76-year expectancy, ranks behind Japan, France, Costa Rica, and the United Kingdom. Increases in chronic diseases such as cardiovascular disease and cancers are being seen in all developing countries, probably the result of extended physical years as much as the influences of technology.

The WHO report examined geographical areas as well. Africa has the most pressing health problems worldwide: poor prevention programs and spreading diseases including meningitis, yellow fever, cholera, plague, malaria, diarrhea, and AIDS.

Asia's infant mortality rates and life expectancy have improved in the past 40 years but many countries are not dealing with "lifestyle diseases" such as heart disease, cancer, drug abuse, and AIDS.

Middle East contends with infectious diseases, and diabetes is beginning to emerge as a serious problem as people change eating habits and lifestyle.

The report concludes that Europeans smoke and drink too much, and must now cope with the reappearance of tuberculosis and diphtheria which scientists believed were under control.

It is astounding to see mankind's evolutionary progress through the eyes of researchers who seek what is wrong about us rather than what is right. This commonplace thinking is the result of man's inner urge to *create*, he just tends to interpret it outwardly as an urge to *correct*. In the future this will change as he realizes more profoundly the power of his own thought.

Rather than a negative view of the world, these statistics are an affirmation of man's continuing progress toward awareness and enlightenment. The different points on the globe and their individual challenges offer the soul a wide variety of learning opportunities upon incarnation. Globally the physical causes of disorders as identified by science give man more individual freedom and responsibility. The mental attitudes which support susceptibility to those disorders reveal a great deal about the commonalities of groups of people no matter where they live on earth.

What these statistics say to me is that for the most part we have as a species moved beyond the responsibility level of the animal, reacting to other life forms, and we have advanced to be the aware and conscious thinker who chooses how he will interact in a world filled with other life forms. Man has learned to cooperate with the elements, taming them. He purifies water so it is drinkable, he builds shelters to moderate temperature, he can even predict dangerous weather so people can temporarily migrate to safer land areas. Nature's violence is less and less a threat to a technologically advanced humanity. Once immunity is built to that which comes from without and is destructive to man, awareness of that which comes from within must be responded to.

This becomes apparent in the report's assessment of health in the Americas where life expectancy is "good" and infant mortality rates low. *But* violence has become a critical public health problem in many large cities.

The U.S. Department of Health supports this conclusion. Among the entries on its leading cause of death list are: number four *"unintentional injuries"* including motor vehicle accidents, number eight *suicide* and number 10 *homicide*. When man no longer needs to fight the elements in his environment, nature's challenges to his health, he comes face-to-face with self-inflicted dangers. At first glance these may appear to be very physical causes of death, but in each case there are mental or emotional factors that are behind the violent deaths. Statistics show over fifty percent of traffic accidents are caused by *inattentiveness*, mental laziness or distraction. Suicides are motivated by real or imagined *fear*. The vast majority of people who commit suicide are running away from life situations they do not want to face. Rather than lose something in life – family or loved ones, financial security, good health – they exit. Most homicides are perpetrated on people the killer knows. People in this country rarely kill strangers, they kill people they have strong attachments to and they kill in moments of *blinding emotion*. Man's acts of violence do not just happen, they are caused. Most violent crimes in the U.S. are domestic, people hurting the people they supposedly love. Since technology has reduced the external threats to our health, mankind finds less opportunity to band with others for survival. The "common enemy" is disappearing. In the near future, man must learn how to cooperate with others, uniting from choice *because everyone will benefit*. He must be willing to live "the golden rule." Violence will be a health hazard until man learns how to cause peace within Self. A Tenton Sioux proverb puts it all together, "Inner peace and love are the greatest of God's gifts." The peace that births wholistic well-being is the real health challenge of the future.

How we meet this challenge will determine whether we move forward quickly to an enlightened age or stumble in the dark prejudices of the past.

Consider this, U.S. and British researchers recently identified regions of the brain that may play a part in why schizophrenics hear voices and see things that don't [physically] exist. By studying six people, they isolated the areas of the brain that are active when a real [physical] voice is heard – the interconnected core and surface regions. The core is associated with thought, emotions, and perceptions while the surface generally processes information such as hearing. During hallucinations more of the core regions are turned on than would be if the person just heard or saw something, reported the study.

One of the researchers from New York Hospital - Cornell Medical Center said, "The overactivity in the core indicates the brain is creating its own reality and believing it." The research suggests new drugs could be used to control the activity of those regions said a professor of psychiatry at Mount Sinai School of Medicine.

Most people's first response to this announcement would be laudatory. How wonderful that man can help these unfortunate people be normal. The arrogance in this way of thinking is lost because it is so widely accepted in our society. Arrogant it is nevertheless. The "dumbing down" in health care is as reprehensible as it in public education. Neither makes society a better place to live. Equalizing in both cases causes society to lose the potential it needs to cultivate the most.

Just when people are beginning to use more of their brain power... Just when people are beginning to tap the vast inner realms of consciousness not dependent upon the physical world and senses... Just when people are beginning to experience mystical Kundalini experiences... Just when you thought it was acceptable to talk about the voices you hear, or angels you see... comes the established "normal" experts with a study and a drug to inhibit and restrict the "abnormality" before even identifying its purpose, function, and possible benefit to the person and to society. Yes, chemicals can be used to bring about a balance, and in the case of an antisocial, unconscionable person their use would be a benefit to all. But to make it seem as though everyone whose brains are more fully functional than the average needs to be medicated, is the thinking of one obsessed with controlling another; the result of small egotistical minds who limit the use of their own brain capacity and seek to do the same to others.

A true researcher will investigate how, when, and why these people can hear and see beyond what is physical so all of us can learn to use more of our brain power. They will manifest science at its highest expression, exploring what man can do. The inner realms of consciousness are where the very real experiences of precognition, telekinetic activity, kundalini arousal, and telepathic connections take place.

This is the new frontier that awaits our investigation and understanding. Let us move forward with the integrity and dignity befitting a Creator's most promising prodigy.

In the not too distant future, the physician will also be a *meta*physician. And we will all be healthier for it.

Part IV

Care in the 21st Century

T here is this difference

between the two temporal blessings – health and money;

money is the most envied, but the least enjoyed;

health is the most enjoyed, but the least envied;

and this superiority of the latter is still more obvious when we

reflect that the poorest man would not part with health for money,

but that the richest would gladly part with all his money for health.

– Caleb Colton, English clergyman, 19th century

T he very success of medicine in a material way

may now threaten the soul of medicine.

Medicine is something more than the cold

mechanical application of science to human disease.

Medicine is a healing art.

It must deal with individuals,

their fears, their hopes and their sorrows.

– Dr. Walter Martin, former AMA president, 20th century

The Future of Health

In the oldest religious scriptures of the world, which are the *Vedas* of India, there is a concept that is very much a part of the Hindu faith. This is known as the pairs of opposites. The pairs of opposites describes a Universal Principle evidenced throughout creation.

When a soul becomes entrapped or engrossed in physical, material existence, it becomes subject to a manifestation of the Universal Law of Duality. That means we are constantly buffeted by what we identify as opposites: hot and cold, sweet and sour, tall and short. We use opposites to identify the physical world around us in order to hopefully identify the meaning of why we are here. The engrossed soul, the person we are outwardly, falls in love with the pairs of opposites. We find ourselves buffeted by opposites: by like and dislike, by pleasure and pain.

School of Metaphysics teachings empower you to understand those opposites and know how to transcend them. This causes something that is revolutionary in the world, and quite controversial. While most of the world's leaders are touting diversity as the way to global cohabitation, we surpass the finite differences finding the point of unity. We encourage, indeed insist that, the diversities of what we find in the physical must be placed in proper perspective. This can only be done when awareness rises above the pairs of opposites to the point of cause. From this point we can truly accept and respect the many expressions which emanate from the source like rays from the sun. By rooting our awareness at this point of origin we know unity in our experiences. We can experience from the level of the soul, rather that from the grosser level of the entrapped physical person.

Metaphysical investigation ultimately frees the individual from entrapment, from being a slave to the five physical senses. The liberated soul sees with new eyes. The liberated soul can recognize other souls. Such a one salutes the divinity in each person, seeing no one as a stranger. For when there is awareness of a common Source, we are all spiritual siblings.

What this kind of thinking produces is a unity of religion and science. This is a revolutionary concept in today's world. You might find this theory elsewhere but in few, if any, places will you find it openly discussed and put into practice.

As we go into the next millennium this will change. It is indeed the future of mankind to realize that science and religion are compatible, the two halves needed to make a whole. They are not opposites and they are not enemies. They are merely paths of knowledge seeking to identify and to explore life.   Both must be present for there to be a complete understanding of any one thing for they represent the uniting of conscious reasoning and subconscious intuition. Both reasoning and intuition must be present for man to realize wholeness.

The Intuitive Health Analyses clear the way for this marriage. So does the extensive research on intuitively-accessed historical information derived from thousands of past lifetime accounts. Those detailing the Atlantean time period are fascinating to most people because there is so little available data on earlier time periods in mankind's evolution.   A greater cause for excitement is what these histories tell us about mankind today.

Apart from Plato's mention of Atlantis in The Republic, few references to the lost continent exist today. Most movable records from the period, or writings concerning it, were lost in the fire which destroyed the Great Library of Alexandria. A few of these were rescued and, from accounts, apparently made their way to the library in Vatican City. For the most part what is written about Atlantis is intuitively-gained knowledge. Accurate information about the people of Atlantis is particularly pertinent to mankind now because, as a race, humankind is experiencing the culmination of what was begun during the Atlantean time period and the initiation of a new stage of evolutionary growth. [Research regarding this is detailed in The Rising of Atlantis and the Emergence of Spiritual Man.] There are several relevant themes that echo from those past times into the present, even though the Atlantean time period centered on the development of reasoning in animal man and the present time period brings a new focus – the evolutionary development of intuition in spiritual man.

Much of what has been perceived and written about the time period has been misinterpreted. Many authors make their impressions sound like horror stories of all manner of aberrations. For example, many assert that mythological characters are not the result of imagination rather they are a description of creatures that once existed. I believe those who hold these ideas perceive inner level energies but misinterpret the time and place for them. In other words, many of the horror stories that are said to have happened in Atlantis, are actually happening today.

The combination of man and animal didn't happen in some distant time in man's past. Rather these happen today. The commonplace material used for skin grafts on burn victims is pigskin. Pigskin is attached to human flesh. What does that make that person? Does it make him part man and part pig? Or consider this, in the last decade of the 1900's the first heart transplant from a baboon to a human being was successfully made. What does that make the physical body? Part baboon, part human, a monkey-man? No more than you becoming that Ford when you get in your car to drive somewhere. But historians could write about the practice in such a way to create a horror story. Or more likely an allegory, a story, of mankind's journey from dark to light, ignorance to wisdom. I believe this to be the essence and import of all mythology.

I also believe many of the so-called Atlantean stories from the past two centuries are not of Atlantis at all but rather glimpses into the future we now are living. They are manifestation of man's reasoning capacity: his experimentations, his attempts to be a creator, his utilization of new and better technology, his attempts to find answers to problems that he sees and many times has created. Some of these attempts, though honestly approached, result in aberrations. Think of the well-intentioned thalidomide of the 1960's that was meant to make the mother-to-be more comfortable by ending the nausea of early pregnancy but produced changes in the growing fetus resulting in deformed babies.

Many of the stories describe what man is now creating in his attempts to maintain good physical health and extend longevity. One of the newest medical technologies involves taking human cells that can be reproduced, in this case the foreskin from circumcised boys, to make skin that then can be used for grafts. Human body parts to human bodies. It is only a matter of time, and the result of the natural progression of man's experimentation, that what was yesterday's imagined fiction becomes today's realized science.

This was profoundly brought home for the world to consider with a Scottish ewe named Dolly. In early 1997, scientists in Scotland announced they had extracted the DNA from one cell of a ewe and placed it on another cell thereby cloning the original. The news ignited global imagination.

It might seem a big jump from sheep to humans but within days of the Scottish announcement came a report that Oregon scientists in the United States had produced a clone of a monkey from an embryo. The question "can our species be far behind?" suddenly jumped off the pages of science fiction for all of us. Everyone had something to say.

"At first glance, we might want to live in a world where there would always be a Gandhi or Lincoln or da Vinci," a rabbi said. "But I think the reality would be living in a world where there would always be a Michael Jackson."

"If we could make a clone from one of Lincoln's hairs," surmised a journalist, "what we might get is a tall man who looks like a five dollar bill. Genius is touched by conscience. Character is not a product of chromosomes. Character is what makes someone worth revering and impossible to reproduce."

A science editor and author observed, "If this technology can be used on humans, it will produce replicas not offspring. Then man will be creating a new class of beings. And that's a scary thought. You might some day be ordering them from a catalogue."

It was not just scientists and theologians who confronted the reality of cloning. People of all professions worldwide now knew of the existing technology that makes human cloning imminently probable. Yet when one of the doctors heading the project was asked about the implications of his work toward human cloning his response was simple, "Why would you want to do that?" Some would argue that because these scientists are experts in livestock breeding, not human morality, they are short-sighted. But I think it's more likely their work enables them to separate humanity from animals more readily than the rest of us thus making them visionaries seeing much farther down the road of probabilities than those who have just begun to think about it.

And think about it we are. Within a day of the announcement of the

Scotland experiment, governmental leaders called for studies and commissions on the legal and ethical issues of cloning, and the possible need for government intervention. Should there be regulation of research? Should government fund research? Animal protection? Should laws making cloning illegal be written? Should the limits be set by local, country, or world standards? These questions have rarely been seriously discussed because cloning was not a reality, now it is.

And of course there is a lawyer's viewpoint: "Any attempt to impede intellectual and scientific progress is a mistake. It's like closing the [U.S.] patent office in the mid-1900's because nothing else should be invented. It was stupid. There's never been a discovery without negative side effects – fire, the wheel, internal combustion engine. The best minds must weigh the good and bad sides of the science, then try to regulate the negative side with laws." It still remains you cannot legislate morality, and perhaps that is what concerns people the most. After all history proves that the best laws are broken by the worst people.

What does it all mean? What will our future be? At the point of every scientific breakthrough, people ask fundamental questions. Metaphysicians recognize four timeless questions: *Where did we come from? Why are we here? Where are we going?* These remain the fundamental questions asked by humanity since the dawn of self-consciousness and the ability to reason. Human cloning directly challenges current answers to the final question: *Who am I?*

Even without benefit of producing physical human clones, scientists will tell you that if you expect that cloned human baby will become a copy of the original, then you will be disappointed. A human clone will not be a replica for a simple reason, a clone will not live the experiences of the original. It can't live the original's life.

At best a clone will be like identical twins who start out genetically the same but over time become distinctly different people. A scientist will say environment counts; it shapes the genes and genes can't reproduce an exact copy of person. The decisions you make today – what to wear, eat, read, say – are not written in your genes. Any mother of twins will gladly tell any scientist the unique expressions, desires, preferences displayed by their children from the day they were born. The soul does not derive its uniqueness from external conditions but rather from what springs from within the being, what comes from the spirit. This is the realm of the metaphysician.

A metaphysician understands the scientific guess that a clone will not be the original because it will not have the original's experiences. This is true in the context of linear space and time, in other words the clone will exist two years or five years or forty years later than the original making his environmental experiences different. But what about his inner experiences? There are vertical time factors that dictate the differences existing at the time of birth, the time of the soul's incarnation. Metaphysicians understand this realm because they are willing to do something scientists have yet to incorporate in their understanding. Metaphysicians are willing to separate the soul from the body, the immortal spirit of who you are from the temporary flesh of what you are. The scientist says cloning will never make anyone immortal. The metaphysician explains why: cloning is the manipulation of matter, not the creation of a soul.

The technological availability of cloning does challenge how we see ourselves and the world. For thousands of years, mankind generally held three concepts as being universally true:

1] Mankind required a female and a male to produce offspring.

2] The offspring wasn't exactly like the mother or the father but a combination of the two.

3] God, or for those without religious conviction the genetic structure, was responsible for selecting among all the options

These concepts are no longer true. The cloning of a female sheep from a female sheep changed these concepts. The spectre of human cloning is more than man playing God. It is a challenge to traditional understanding of our universe because now *we are our own creators*.

Humanity has been "playing God" for centuries. From the ancient Chinese herbs that produced immunity to the Hebrew handmaids who bore children for their mistresses to manmade bionic limbs, man has always found a way to fulfill his physical desires. The inherent urge that propels him is maturity, a spiritual need to be like his Creator. In this context is it so strange to believe that man would also want to create in *his* image? This is exactly what he does.

It required thousands of years before mankind developed sufficient understanding of procreation that pregnancy could be avoided through altering the chemical balance in the female body – the birth control pill of the 1960's. This produced the so-called sexual revolution. Although women had created many ways to avoid childbearing "the pill" was by far the easiest and the most reliable. Its use alleviated fears that each sexual contact might lead to pregnancy. What had been the domain of God or genetic law was now in human hands.

Cloning is the natural last step of a series steps in mankind's desire to plan families according to his own will. Technology has revealed man as a creator: *in vitro* fertilization, surrogate pregnancies, test tube babies. Science has enabled anyone to make their own children, one way or another. Up until now, science's role has been seen as helping nature. Technology has been concerned with the basic fundamental principle of reproduction. Now, however, we are talking about replication. This is very different. The potential is no longer to aid nature, to cooperate with what exists, but to bring into existence something apart from nature. Man is no longer playing, he is serious about being God.

The ultimate question might really be, if man does create human clones will there be souls willing to inhabit those bodies? The more immediate lesson of human cloning will involve the pairs of opposites, beginning with the separation of body and soul. The classic philosophical question of human cloning involves hypothetical parents who lose a 4-year-old child. Will they want to take a swab from that child's gums and make a clone? At best the clone would be a replacement child. Cloning will not give relief of the sorrow for no one can replace the lost child. A physical replica may look like the lost child but the clone would be another child with its own distinct experiences. More accurately, in order for the clone-body to live, a soul will need to commit to using that body.

From our research into these realms it is unlikely that a soul who has just departed the physical world will immediately return to inhabit another body. Man may indeed be accelerating as a physical creator but he still lacks the wisdom to clone the soul. Perhaps it is the issue of cloning that will compel man's spiritual maturity to catch up with his physical capabilities. Afterall, cloning humans does in all probability mean that females will no longer require males to reproduce. The possibility of mass production of cloned babies, quality controlled for potential disease, better looking, stronger, takes selective breeding out of nature's hands and places the responsibility in man's hands. If man wants the freedom to choose he had better be prepared to accept the responsibility for his choice.

This has repeatedly been the pair of opposites challenging man as a reasoner: freedom and responsibility. This is the latest societal Pandora's box. The temptation is the same as it has always been with scientific research and technological development: "Just imagine what good can come of it!" If you're skeptical of scientists' motives, examine your own. Averaging several media polls here's how the layman views it:

Do you approve of cloning in scientific research?
Yes 39%   **No 50%**

Do you approve of cloning for medical research?
Yes 53%   No 43%

Do you approve of cloning humans?
Yes 10%   **No 87%**

Would you want to personally be cloned?
Yes 6%   **No 93%**

The one area where society can be persuaded to accept human cloning is *medical research*. The real question is just because we can, should we? The medical applications are profound. This is the part that will in all likelihood motivate us on.

The probability is that human cloning is going to happen. Commercial and political pressures will find benefit in it, pursue it, and accomplish it. Twenty years ago *in vitro* fertilization was science fiction, done only in laboratories and experiments. Now you can obtain the procedure through most Health Maintenance Organizations. This will be the story of cloning unless those who pursue the work can transcend it, thus tempering their own experiments with enlightened conscience.

We must ask, "when should science end and moral values take over in deciding progress?" This is a basic cultural question. It becomes a matter of public debate, something for society to consider. The real concern is that the whole concept of experimentation is technology-driven. The thinking person knows just because you can, doesn't mean you do. Unfortunately in science the license is usually taken, and so when they can, they do.

Mankind stands at the threshold of a spiritual maturity. Will he remain a rebellious adolescent, insisting upon going through every experience conceivable finding his wisdom in hindsight alone? Or will he listen to reason, channeling his powerful imagination to perceive lines of probability before committing mind and body to a series of actions. Do we as a species have the moral fiber and illumined conviction to say no to technology?

When all is said and done any attempt to outlaw cloning will represent the current consensus to slow down. Cloning animals is such a simple procedure there is no reason to think cloning the human body will be any different. Government can not police the activity, but government could punish. And like Pandora once the box is opened, the spirits unleashed must be tamed.

It is too late for a ban on cloning. The procedure is known to have been done at several points around the globe and probably several more we don't know about. To keep cloning in a research mode for a long time where experiments can be carefully monitored and regulated will be the agreement of honorable and reasonable people. Most of the world's leaders will realize we have to take the lead or technology will run away and we will have uncontrolled human cloning.

Senior writer John Horgan of *Scientific American* put the technology into perspective when he noted, "Science...has given us vaccines and birth control pills and jets and laptop computers. But we still cannot comprehend ourselves. We still get cancer and become depressed. We still grow old and diet. Far from becoming God-like, we are as mortal as ever."

When all is said and done, humanity will survive cloning not by manmade law but by ripened reason. This is not the first time science has risked destruction. The potential has existed for decades in man's control of nuclear energy. When Hiroshima occasioned anxious talk about the dangers of physics, Albert Einstein replied that the world was more apt to be destroyed by bad politics than by bad physics. Keep in mind it is sameness that eventually makes a species extinct.

Science is the pursuit of what man *can do* while theology is the quest for what man *ought to do*. The reality of man's experimentation as a creator is that responding to what man can do requires both the avid curiosity of the scientist and the divine inspiration of the saint. Science and religion must do more than talk, more than cooperate, science and religion must unite and become one. It will require this melding to produce the enlightenment necessary to respond to the temptation of cloning humans in the hope of curing physical disease.

The revolution has begun. And we must mature our thinking to guide it into an acceleration of spiritual evolution. The need for wisdom is great. The responsibility for our future lies with those who are directly involved in man's creative endeavors but no less so upon each of our shoulders. We must be committed to expanding our awareness. We must be willing to release attachment to those pairs of opposites. That attachment is pronounced in the spiritual, mental, emotional and physical condition of the individual.

Unite religious and science and you find a perfect blend right here and now of what man is capable of doing in this stage of his evolution. Remain attached to diversity, the differences in intent or approach or even outcome, and the two pull apart taking their stances in opposition. We miss the point becoming further entrapped in the pairs of opposites. When health is the issue this means the differences between wellness and disease, recovery and decline, life and death.

So you find people who always go the medical route. They have a pain so they go to a doctor and the doctor prescribes a drug. Soon the body builds a tolerance to the drug; it no longer alters the symptoms. A greater concentration is prescribed or a substitute drug is given. One drug leads to another drug and another, each with its own unique side effects. The patient may want to stop "medication" but is insecure or fearful of the effects when he does. He is now addicted to drugs. His body now belongs to science. He is dependent upon artificial chemicals to alter his body's natural chemistry so he is no longer aware of his body's attempts to alert him that something is wrong. Because there is no faith, there is no religion, there is no belief that there can be a change in the physical condition without medical technology.

By the same token you have probably heard stories about people who refused allopathic treatment on the basis of their religious beliefs even when the problem is life-threatening and proven treatments exist. They absolutely refuse what science has to offer, almost as if it didn't exist. Sometimes they get better and sometimes they die. In this day and age unnecessarily.

Two extremes. One adhering only to religion, the other only to medical technology. Each are not satisfying because alone they do not produce what we want ideally which is a whole and healthy condition. This becomes the challenge of today. How we meet it will determine society's awareness tomorrow.

The challenge makes demands on each of us. It requires us to explore possibilities, to think beyond immediate needs into the probabilities of the future. It requires us to release prejudices, opening our consciousness so we might think as a soul with a body rather than a body that hopefully has a soul, somewhere.

I have had a wealth of experience in this lifetime. Each has led me to these visions of the future. For the first twelve years of my life our household included my parents, me, and my grandparents. This was significant because my grandfather was a Christian evangelist. He was a faith healer. He would place his hands on those wanting healing, often on the diseased part of the body. He prayed that he might be a channel for God's healing power so it might flow through him and into this individual to heal their physical body. He always gave God the credit and never himself. Whatever the source of the power, all manners of illnesses, everything from crossed-eyes to limps to alcoholism, left.

Some healings I witnessed, others I heard or read about. An account most pronounced in my memory involved a deformed baby. The child's hands were malformed, they had not opened since birth. The fingers not only curled in toward the palm of the hand but they were sealed together appearing to be one continuous unit making the hands resemble claws. The child was a year or two old when his mother brought him to my grandfather. Grandfather laid hands on the child, and people could see the healing occur. Immediately the skin connecting the child's fingers separated and he was able to move the now independent digits.

This is the power of faith. Such miraculous healings have been a part of my life since birth. When young, if I was sick from a stomachache or earache, my mother didn't reach for aspirin or an over-the-counter medicine. Rather she would take me to my grandfather, sometimes in the middle of the night, and he would pray for me. Every time he prayed for me I felt better.

Now I understand more what caused the healing. It was a combination of factors: my belief in my grandfather, his talent and skill, and his belief in God, a greater power that would cause healing when called upon. The core was the faith; the faith that there could indeed be a change. Miraculous healing, no matter when it is accomplished or by whom, requires this kind of pure, unadulterated belief. Faith that through some power there can be a transformation, there can be an entire change from illness to wholeness, from feeling bad to feeling good. Every time this faith is present healing occurs.

Since then I have pursued learning, seeking to understand the whys to what I see and hear. I try to keep abreast of significant studies by all manners of professionals at colleges and universities around the world. Such information lets me know what man is doing as a creator, what technologies he is developing. I think it is most important, particularly in the areas of health and healing, that we utilize everything available to us. That means that we must investigate and learn how to harness the power of our minds. We must learn to respect the mental action of faith realizing that the way we construct thinking sets into motion effects or consequences. We must accept the fact that mankind, whether it is us personally or someone else, has used his talent and genius to fashion all types of technologies in an attempt to learn how to be a creator. Technologies that we now are individually *and* collectively responsible for.

With technology, health has moved away from being an individual challenge of faith and fortitude to being big business where millions of peoples' jobs depend upon sick people who want to be well. The health industry in the United States of America is *one-seventh* of the economy of our country. Think about all the businesses you use during the day, from where you purchase the gas for your car to the restaurant where you eat or the grocery store where you purchase food to the shops where you buy your clothes to the cleaners who launder them to your own business or place of employment to even the contractors who build the buildings. Think of all these different industries, all the ways that people are employed in the United States today. Take one-seventh of that; that is how much of our society is involved in the health industry. This is a huge part of our economy. Beyond the financial implications, it speaks volumes about ourselves for this percentage reflects our consciousness as a society. One-seventh of the consciousness of our nation is interested in, committed to, consumed by, and invested in the pursuit of good health.

You would expect U.S. citizens to be the healthiest people on the planet. But we aren't. There are so many luxuries to living in this country, in spite of the picture often painted by a ratings-profit driven media, no one in this country need ever go to sleep hungry or without a roof over their heads. The U.S. has the highest percentage of volunteerism in the world, people helping people. The U.S. problem does not lie in battling the elements. The U.S. problem lies in battling sloth. The wealthiest nation on earth faces the same challenges wealthy individuals have always faced, when physical needs are easily met how do you remain viable? The fruits of the wealth must be used wisely, never taken for granted, lest the mind be wasted, the spirit ignored, and the body abused from overindulgences.

The truth is we have yet to learn how to respond productively as individuals and as a society to our wealth. Technology is virtually replacing the need for manual labor. From backhoes that dig ditches and graves to automatic screwdrivers, living no longer makes demands upon the physical body that once kept it toned and vibrant. At the same time, we find an endless supply of food, from fast food to all-you-can-eat restaurants to grocers who stock every food available on the planet, waiting to be consumed. We are fast becoming a society of gluttons, consuming much more than we require. It is what the rest of the world criticizes us for, and they are right. We may be giddy with wealth now but when one day you awake to find your mind dulled by alcohol or drugs or food that has fermented in your body, and your body weakened and diseased, you may find all your wealth being used in an effort to restore personal dignity and physical health. First things first. As Ralph Waldo Emerson observed, "The first wealth *is* health."

Too many people have to lose before they appreciate. Those who earn something in life tend to prize what they have more highly than those who are given something without paying for it. The imagination, will, and attentive effort required to create and fulfill desires brings an understanding of value. Most people have to go through a physically debilitating experience before they are sufficiently motivated to pursue good health. For some the stimulus required for change can seem too simple: a toothache which makes eating painful or a few extra pounds on the scales. For others the stimulus is much more dramatic. It takes more to get their attention: a migraine headache so blinding that to move causes paralyzing pain or a spinal misalignment that makes walking impossible. When you have taken the functioning of your body for granted, you are shocked when it fails you.

How you respond to the loss determines the future of your health.

Respecting what you have is the root of all wealth. The family poor in material possessions is often the wealthiest spiritually from necessity. The true challenge for mankind now and in the future is how to increase the spirit midst a richness of material possessions. We must transcend our own limitations, going beyond the least line of resistance which is to be material creators. We must learn to be spiritual creators. This is most true in the area of health. For example, throughout the last half of the 1900's science was looking for a replacement for sugar, commonly derived from sugar cane. The first manmade chemical replacement was saccharin. It enjoyed a widespread popularity until long term tests indicated saccharin might contribute to cancer at which time the Federal Drug Agency took the substance off the open market. It wasn't too many years until a new chemical, aspartame, was invented and is now enjoying popularity as an artificial sweetener in everything from soft drinks to canned fruits to breads. Now that some years of use have passed, studies on aspartame indicate that the chemical is not particularly healthy for the body either. Being an artificial substance it is not assimilated by the body and so becomes a toxic substance stored in the liver. There are cases where aspartame has been shown to contribute to nervous disorders and liver disease as well as aggravating preexisting conditions. Man's original intention may be to help – let's produce something that tastes good but is not caloric – but any time he seeks to cure an effect he just sets into motion more difficulties. Look at the lengthy description of possible side effects to any drug on the market and you will see the report card for man as a creator.

We must learn to go beyond appearances, beyond material wealth, beyond what sounds good. Your *wholistic* health makes your life a happy treasure or a miserable waste. The more you know about spirit, mind, and body, the more intelligent your choices. And in this day of quick fixes – artificial chemicals in foods, symptom masking drugs – to have control of your physical health you must become knowledgeable about what exists. When I was pregnant with my son, my chiropractor suggested a fiber product to help ease the distress on the alimentary system. The next few mornings I mixed a bit with juice and found it produced the desired effect. By the end of the week, I noticed the drink was what I thought unnecessarily sweet so I read the label. I expected to find all natural ingredients, like psyllium seed husks, acidophilous, or apple pectin. I got much more than

I bargained for, far down the list of natural ingredients was "aspartame". I had read quite a bit about diet during pregnancy, particularly chemical additives in processed foods and aspartame was in most of the books I read. The jury was out, nobody really knew what aspartame does to the human body much less a growing fetus so the books recommended avoiding it during pregnancy. I stopped using the product and looked for one with all natural ingredients.

We become so attached to quickness, so attached to having what we want when we want it, to things being easy, that we forgo our command of being able to create health in our physical body. Every time we look for convenience or quickness we are giving up some kind of freedom. Every time you consume a product with a large percentage of man-made chemicals – those strange words on the label that you don't understand – remember this: you are putting stresses on your physical body that *the body was never meant to have.* Keep in mind these chemicals are the result of man's technology. Many were created for commercial appeal. Some were created to increase the shelf life, to make the product last longer before it deteriorates. Just imagine what those kind of chemicals do inside your body! If a chemical preserves a living substance beyond its natural life span so you can eat it, it probably will not extend its consumer's life span but rather make whatever nutrition available difficult to assimilate. Just because man can create it does not necessarily mean that it is health-producing for you.

It has only been in the last fifty years that cancer has become the number one killer in the United States. Before that it was heart disease. Statistics tend to credit technology that enables surgery, cleansing of arteries, even transplants to replaced diseased hearts as the reason for decrease in heart disease deaths. It is probably also true that the credit for the rise in cancers belongs to technology that has ensured we are exposed to chemical compounds not normally found in nature. Daily exposure to these chemicals in food, water, and air tax the body. From the chemicals that clean the clothes we wear to those used in the houses we live in, most of us, particularly city dwellers, live in artificial environments that the body must adapt to. No doubt genetic changes are resulting from constant exposure, and no doubt constant exposure is disrupting previously normal, functioning cells.

There is a quote in the Bible that comes back to me each time I think about man's efforts to control his life through technology, "The road to hell is paved with good intentions." This pretty much summarizes mankind's attempts to be a creator in the 1900's. It epitomizes the pairs of opposites because for every ill there is a cure, for every good there is an evil. This is the nature of the physical. This natural law of balance is the physical expression of a Universal Law, Cause and Effect. Anything that can be created by man can have a productive use. It can also be turned around and have a destructive use. It depends not upon the creation itself but upon the creative intelligence using the creation. Atomic energy is wonderful. It is used to power lights and to regulate the temperature in rooms where we live. Atomic energy can also be used to instantly kill thousands of people. Pesticides can kill plant eating bugs thereby yielding more food for human consumption or it can sink into the water table contaminating human water supplies making it unfit to drink. Motor vehicles are wonderful inventions that enable us to travel at will but in the hands of alcohol-dulled drivers they become weapons.

Everything always comes back to the mind of man, his maturity and level of responsibility. What is your state of awareness, what is your intention in everything you do? Your state of health spiritually in many ways dictates your mental, emotional and physical health.

In the near future, man will undergo a change in motivation from the immediate sensual gratification to the purposeful thinking that leads to fulfillment. The present "save the earth" organizations are one expression of this shift in consciousness. So are recycling efforts. So is the overwhelming popularity of natural remedies: herbs, vitamins, and other health foods. People who create the products we use will demonstrate a vision never before seen. Choices will be made based upon what is going to happen in ten or twenty years. This will necessitate a unity of philosophy and science, the utilization of reasoning and intuition.

I remember that when I was very young a lot of the religious people around me were very suspicious of doctors. They were reluctant to seek medical care even when in great pain. Such action was interpreted as a weakness of faith. Throughout my lifetime I have seen a change in attitude, an openness. Now many religious people believe God put doctors on earth to help us. They believe God calls certain people to be doctors, to help do his work. This is an excellent example of religion uniting with science.

What is exciting to me is that soon we are going to see a similar kind of openness happening on the scientific side. Traditionally, scientists do not want anything they are doing tainted with the *super*natural. Furthermore when dealing with medical science, physicians can be intimidated by what they don't know making them slow to change. However some phenomenally open-minded physicians are paving the way for the union of science with the religious. In addition to the reknown Deepak Chopra, there are many physicians pioneering their own field. Dr. Bernie Seigel and Dr. Andrew Weil are both medical doctors and authors of best-selling books, and <u>Peace</u>, <u>Love</u>, and <u>Healing</u> and <u>Spontaneous</u> <u>Healing</u> respectively. Lesser known but more substantial in the future potential of what is he contributing is Dr. Norman Shealy. Dr. Shealy began as a neurosurgeon, graduated to pain control without drugs and now is developing ways to regenerate tissue. His research is phenomenal, results astounding, reflecting the future of wholistic medical care.

Hopefully the future of wholistic health care will continue to be shaped by SOM research. Our headquarters is located on 1500 acres of beautiful countryside in southern Missouri where we plan to build a four-year college teaching the arts and sciences from the soul's point of view. Part of the dream is a Wholistic Health & Healing Center where those in need can come to replenish the spirit, rejuvenate the mind, and heal the body. Upon your arrival you will receive an Intuitive Health Analysis. We want to help people create wholistic health. What makes something wholistic is understanding a cause for every element that makes up the whole. Therefore the spiritual, mental, emotional, and physical needs must first be identified. The health analysis becomes a first opinion. Once the analysis is received a certified psi counselor, who knows how to use both conscious and subconscious minds, will aid the client to resolve pressures that wound the psyche. Classes in positive thinking will empower people to replace old, defeatist patterns of thinking with expansive, innovative ideas. Experts in dream interpretation will teach them to use their dreams to accelerate the healing process. These will guide the client to deeper levels of understanding the origin of his distress and freeing his consciousness from limitation. As the client progresses he will learn how to use his mind to heal himself, and be the recipient of healing energy daily while at the spa.

While the inner self is nurtured, the outer self will be treated to all manners of physical treatments to reestablish healthy functioning. Nutritionists and naturopaths will design a healthful diet including any foods, herbs, or vitamins recommended in the analysis. Chefs will teach how to use these for the optimum health benefit. Recreational and physical therapists will specifically design programs for each client based upon the individual needs. Professional masseurs will ease muscle tension, acupuncturists will free energy flows, chiropractors will realign body structure, and homeopaths will stimulate balance in body chemistry. Should allopathic care be recommended in the analysis, referrals to medical specialists will be given. Wholistic health care. The person who comes here will experience healing. Whether their stay is a weekend, a week, or a month, what they can hope to gain is a transformation of how they look at themselves, how they look at life, and how they look at health. The Wholistic Health & Healing Center is going to be the epitome of achieving health, a prototype that I hope will be reproduced again and again around the world.

Simultaneously, the wholistic education offered at the College of Metaphysics will teach people of all ages and walks of life, from any culture and country on Earth, how to accelerate their spiritual evolution. Through a combination of the applied study in the laws that govern creation, courses in the traditional arts and sciences, and a community of people dedicated to living as Spiritual, Intuitive Man, this college will prepare generations to meet the responsibilities of man as a creator. The effects of maturing reasoning and intuition will be far reaching. Spiritual Man will be a wholistic creator, using everything to its fullest and wasting nothing. His model will be creation, where nothing is ever made new or completely destroyed, only changed in form. And one of the most profound alterations in form will occur as the direct result of becoming Spiritual Man.

One of the founding members of the School of Metaphysics, Dr. Geraldine DeMate Hatcher, shared her excitement and her keen interest in watching our son Hezekiah grow because of the genetics involved in his being here. What she meant was that both my husband and I have been independently pursuing enlightenment through spiritual disciplines for two decades. When you meditate every day for twenty years it causes a change in your consciousness, a change in the vibratory pattern of your being which then affects your physical body.

Let me give you an example of this. Periods of daily meditation nourish the individual in a comparable fashion to the way that daily sleep period nourish the mind and body. Apart from resting the body, sleep allows a replenishing of depleted mental and emotional energies. This is why sleep deprivation can produce everything from mental scatteredness to hallucinations, emotional edginess to hysteria. The very process of creating, visualization, requires intelligence, energy, and substance from the inner mind. Currently man is not taught how to recycle this internal energy source and so must rely upon Universal Laws and genetics to supply it while he unconsciously sleeps. The meditator begins to take control of this automatic ability. The action of meditation stimulates the mind's recycling centers known as chakras which is why meditation refreshes the mental outlook. Meditation periods also have the same physiological benefits as naps. Most importantly, meditation when the intent is communion with the Creator enriches the spirit by elevating consciousness. Meditating for years causes the meditative state to be integrated into your consciousness.

The same is true of consciously calling upon your creative energy, known as Kundalini in Eastern literature. Repeated use alters consciousness. The individual becomes more proficient in reasoning and displays improved intuitive faculties. These uses of human potential change the structure of the human brain. They accelerate nerve impulses affecting the way brain patterns are formed. Increased activity causes an enlargement of the pineal gland and the release of melatonin. It also causes an enlargement of the pituitary gland and the release of endorphins. The heartbeat slows, as energy is removed from the trunk of the body and directed to the brain. Ultimately breathing is slowed and eventually a breathless state can be achieved. These are some of the physical changes that occur within the individual who is developing his consciousness in ways most people only dream about.

With these identifiable changes in the body it is reasonable to expect progressive change in the genetic code. The question is does the expanded consciousness arising through spiritual disciplines encode themselves in the genetic pattern of the aspirant? We believe they do. If this is true, then the uniting of genetics between two such aspirants would potentially create a new kind of body with an innovative genetic structure displaying far more active potential than your average normal structure.

I believe this more than any other future probability will bring about the kind of revelation worthy of the millennium. Until this last century most spiritual knowledge, esoteric teachings of man's relationship to God, has been passed on in secret societies, and most of those are religious; Catholic cardinals, Buddhist monks. Most of them require celibacy as a means of controlling carnal urges that arise from stimulated creative energy. This reflects humanity's immature understanding of Kundalini. Until now man has believed that if you are going to use Kundalini to know God then you must channel that energy up the spine toward the highest spiritual awareness. Channeling the energy downward into the gonads was viewed as a waste of the energy and a reinforcement of physical desire and attachment. There is truth to this thinking but it does not mean that directing Kundalini out into the physical to reproduce the species is a misuse or even a lesser use of the energy. After all, even priests and monks chose bodies from the available genetic pool. For humanity as a race to evolve, spiritually advanced beings must produce offspring. The way we think, the way we live our lives, can produce a genetic pool that is more evolved, more refined, more spiritually inclined.

I had realized many of the differences it would make because Daniel and I had our first child at the beginning of our fourth decade of experiencing. I knew the differences in my consciousness at twenty years of age and my consciousness at forty-one. But I had not brought it all the way out to consider the differences this would mean genetically for the soul who would use the body we created. This, much more than the possibility of cloning, is the future of humanity's development. Love, joy, peace, generosity, goodwill, integrity, honor, respect, dignity, flourish in the evolved conscience. Where these live, no dis-ease can arise. Changes in genetics arise from transformations in consciousness, the maturing of spirit, not from physical manipulations in a laboratory. They will not be the result of a scientific announcement, thrust upon us as a topic for public debate over which we actually have no control. With advancements in understanding we can expect to be prepared to meet the challenges of what we create for they will be a natural outgrowth of who we are.

And who we want to become.

Epilogue

The Truth
is Older than Any of Us

e who has health, has hope;

and he who has hope, has everything.

– Arabian Proverb

The Truth is Older than Any of Us

Each of us is a union of spirit, mind, and body.

Each of us yearn to be whole, compete, at peace.

Each of us possesses the capacity to heal, to cause the fulfillment of desire.

We see the world as we are taught to live it. What we are taught from birth shapes the way we think. As adults we can cause our learning with deeper awareness. This ensures that we teach our offspring from wisdom not limitation. We can build upon our understanding of Universal Truth until we fully realize who we are.

The freedom of self-examination is a recent development in man's evolution. Self-revelation brings us closer to wholeness and well-being which finds its greatest expression in happiness. In his *Meditations* c. 170 Marcus Aurelius said, *"Happiness is, literally, god within, or good."* The happiness we know arises not from the experiences we create in our minds but in the attitude we form about those experiences.

In earlier time periods, the thought of happiness was a luxury. For most people happiness was something to look forward to when the present existence passed away. Thus concepts of a joy-filled afterlife exist in every culture on earth. Before modern inventions and technological innovations, the challenges and dangers of physical survival required constant vigilance. Even now happiness is not a priority in underdeveloped or authoritarian countries where survival is a daily quest.

Those who can afford the thought of happiness have traditionally been the aristocracy, souls incarning in the wealthiest ruling class. Yet let us remember that the life of luxury has its own survival challenges, remember Louis XVI and Marie Antoinette or Czar Nicholas and his wife Alexandria. However, with physical wealth does come the freedom from — freedom from daily toil in the fields or mines or waters or kitchens. Although freedom from can lessen the wear and tear upon the body, it does not necessarily ease the stress and strain upon the mind. Freedom from does not bring happiness. Freedom to can.

How ironic that many of us living in the most prosperous nation on the Earth, the beneficiaries of labor-saving technology, find happiness so elusive. A dwindling middle class accentuates this problem. A small percentage of the middle class has fallen into poverty, becoming part of the lowest class of people. Until the last 50 years of this century, people in the community — neighbors — took care of the poor in their towns. Wealthier families took people into their homes, offering them food and shelter in return for service. Priests and ministers fed the hungry and housed the homeless. Storeowners offered people "having a hard time" jobs equal to their ability. Neighbors would band together to build a new house for a family who lost theirs in a fire. Those who had [the "haves"] made sure others [the "have nots"] also had, and in the process both people discovered happiness as a result of human kindness. A tenet of happiness — close personal relationships — was fulfilled.

However, in recent decades in the U.S. almost all of the poor class have been taught to depend upon government for assistance in housing, feeding and clothing the body, and health care. The happiness which comes from receiving kindness freely given has been usurped by the anger inherent in taking from someone else what does not belong to you. Financial dependency upon something outside of yourself is incongruous with the freedom that comes from earning your own way. This is true for a 16-year-old adolescent standing at adulthood's door but still living under his parents' roof, and for a 42-year-old mother who relies on government for her "welfare". The sense of being in control of one's life, another tenet of happiness, eludes them both. As the Buddhist teachings of 2500 years ago counsel, *"It is good to tame the mind, which is difficult to hold in and flighty, rushing wherever it listeth; a tamed mind brings happiness."*

Likewise those who provide the money for the government to

distribute fail to know the happiness and joy that comes from giving because they are separated from the action. The joy of giving is no longer in their hands. Their contributions are now taxes, their neighbors may never benefit, and someone they don't know does the giving. For all of its high-minded good-intentioned theory, socialization of government violates both tenets of happiness for it weakens the will power that brings self-respect and self-discipline and it destroys opportunities for growth through our relations with others. In reality, governmental socialization has not ended poverty nor has it brought happiness. It has fostered enmity between the classes, driving wedges of fear, resentment, and selfishness between neighbors. The challenges and dangers of survival now come not from wild animals or mother nature but from our own kind. This is the karmic debt of a society that promotes negativity in its citizens.

Most of the middle class has moved upward, as evidenced by bigger homes with two-car garages in classier suburbs with better schools and larger malls. In the back of their minds they believe that a new car, a nanny, a high profile promotion will make them happy. And perhaps it does, for a while. Pursuing happiness is an obsession for many Westerners existing in this high-tech material age. In 370 B.C. Plato wrote, *"Happiness is gained by a use, the right use, of the things of life, and the right use of them, and good-fortune in the use of them is given by knowledge."* And this gives us pause to consider what the 19th century has brought us. While it has made conversation with loved ones as easy as picking up a telephone it has also encouraged us to live physically separated from family members. While it has placed a man on the moon it has also produced millions of tons of manmade waste much of which is toxic. While it has introduced people around the globe to each other through instantaneous televised broadcast of events, it has also fostered mankind's negative self-image through repeated exposure to cruelties inconceivable in the minds of decent men and women.

While technology has brought the world into your home through a computer terminal, it has increased the mental and emotional distance between neighbors and even those living in your own household. Not so long ago when you wanted to learn something you talked to your mom or dad during dinner, or you met with a teacher after school, or you asked your librarian for help. Not so long ago when your car broke down, you went next door to ask your neighbor for a ride to work. Not so long ago a filling station was not just a place to fill your car's gas tank, it was a service station where someone smiled at you, cleaned your windshield so driving would be easier and safer, and offered to check your oil. Not so long ago men opened doors for ladies, young people said "yes, sir" and "no, ma'am", and people knew the neighbors up and down the street by first and last name. Some say this is an ideal world, as if it does not and never did exist. These cynics are pessimists, ever-eager to believe the worst, and so they cast their own destiny.

People who live in a gracious world are well aware that happiness is a frame of mind. They are optimists who believe there is a reason for everything in Heaven and on Earth. Such optimism is the soul of the freedom to that brings happiness to anyone, at any time, anywhere. These people realize happiness inspired by a physical possession or situation can only be fleeting, for by its very nature anything of the physical is constantly changing. The truth is older than any of us. Centuries before the birth of Jesus, Aristotle wrote, *"True happiness flows from the possession of wisdom and virtue and not from the possession of external goods."* This kind of person has had an awakening of the heart and mind to the true origin of happiness. He [or she] dreams of a better life. He trusts. He cares. He treats people as he would have them treat him.

Such a person knows technology, like money, doesn't kill happiness any more than it brings it. Neither does technology or money bring good health. However happiness does promote the well-being that nourishes wholistic health. Science will tell you a happy mind stimulates the endorphins in the brain thus producing the feeling of elation. Thousands of years before science learned this, the Bible offered a prescription for health: *"A cheerful heart is good medicine."*

The root of happiness is found in the Spirit. And when the Spirit is free to manifest its true nature, happiness abounds. He has unlimited faith, believing whole-heartedly in his Maker and in his fellow man. He understands the words of Goethe because he lives them:

"I believe in God—this is a fine, praise-worthy thing to say.
But to acknowledge God wherever and however he manifests
himself, that in truth is heavenly bliss on earth."

About the Author

Born in New Orleans and reared in Missouri, Barbara Condron has served as an educator throughout her adult life. After earning a Bachelors of Journalism degree from the University of Missouri, she pursued her urge for spiritual knowledge through applied studies in metaphysics with the School of Metaphysics. Since earning all degrees offered by that not-for-profit educational institute, Dr. Condron has continued her association with the School in a wide range of positions and responsibilities as a way to serve the growing needs of humanity for spiritual enlightenment. In recognition of her varied accomplishments she is a biographee in Who's Who in America and the World's Who's Who of Women. A minister in the Interfaith Church of Metaphysics, Dr. Condron presented a seminar on *Spiritual Initiation: Gateways to Transcendent Consciousness* during the 1993 Parliament of the World's Religions held in Chicago. Whether teaching, lecturing, or writing about the development of man's potential as a creator, she has stimulated thousands to open their minds and hearts to greater Self awareness. Dr. Condron teaches on the campus of the College of Metaphysics, where she lives with her husband Daniel, also a teacher, author, and administrator for the School of Metaphysics, and their son Hezekiah.

More About *Intuitively-Accessed Information*

Through years of concentration and meditation practices, individuals have reached deeper and deeper states of consciousness. Lucid dreaming, psi development, intuitive skills, and accumulated wisdom are experienced within these inner levels of awareness. Here exists memory that extends beyond the boundaries of physical time and reaches into Man's history, collectively and individually. Here we find the energies that produce well-being and health or dis-ease and sickness.

The intuitively-accessed information available through the School of Metaphysics is the result of years of experimentation in the use of the inner mind to produce insights into states of consciousness and being. Many people find these "readings" reminiscent of Edgar Cayce's work, a Midwesterner who found he possessed a very real psychic ability which was shared with several hundred people during the early part of the 1900's. It is not chance that during the final quarter of this century, again out of the Midwestern United States, comes a very real intuitive ability which has been refined into a skill that can be honed and developed by not just one person, but many.

In addition to the Intuitive Health Analysis, the School can provide an intuitive assessment of soul progression and karmic indenture through three different types of Past Life profiles. These are the subject of the book, *The Work of the Soul*. Intuitively-accessed information is a part of the Spiritual Initiation Weekends offered seven times a year at the Moon Valley Ranch on the College of Metaphysics campus. Except for the sessions described here, these analyses and profiles are given exclusively under the guidance of a mentor who aids you to fully draw upon the wisdom and begin incorporating it into your life.

Research continues in refining and developing areas to assist others in greater understanding of Self through this innovative service. Currently, research is being conducted in the deepest levels of consciousness. These intuitive reports will transcend the soul, going beyond karmic indentures, and revealing the wisdom which wells up from the individual's Spirit. They will hopefully enable the recipient to perceive his highest Self, his Atman, his inner Christ consciousness or Buddha consciousness. In this way we hope to accelerate the evolution and Spiritual Enlightenment of everyone on the planet.

Additional titles available from SOM Publishing include:

The Dreamer's Dictionary
Dr. Barbara Condron ISBN 0944386-16-4 $15.00

The Work of the Soul
Dr. Barbara Condron, ed. ISBN 0944386-17-2 $13.00

Uncommon Knowledge
Past Life & Health Readings
Dr. Barbara Condron, ed. ISBN 0944386-19-9 $13.00

The Universal Language of Mind
The Book of Matthew Interpreted
Dr. Daniel R. Condron   ISBN 0944386-15-6 $13.00

Permanent Healing
Dr. Daniel R. Condron   ISBN 0944386-12-1 $13.00

Dreams of the Soul
The Yogi Sutras of Patanjali
Dr. Daniel R. Condron   ISBN 0944386-11-3 $9.95

Kundalini Rising
Mastering Your Creative Energies
Dr. Barbara Condron ISBN 0944386-13-X $13.00

Shaping Your Life
The Power of Creative Imagery
Laurel Fuller Clark ISBN 0944386-14-8 $9.95

Going in Circles
Our Search for a Satisfying Relationship
Dr. Barbara Condron ISBN 0944386-00-8 $5.95

What Will I Do Tomorrow? Probing Depression
Dr. Barbara Condron ISBN 0944386-02-4 $4.95

Who Were Those Strangers in My Dream?
Dr. Barbara Condron ISBN 0944386-08-3 $4.95

Discovering the Kingdom of Heaven
Dr. Gayle B. Matthes ISBN 0944386-07-5 $5.95

To order write:

School of Metaphysics
World Headquarters
HCR 1, Box 15
Windyville, Missouri 65783
U.S.A.

Enclose a check or money order payable in U.S. funds to SOM with any order. Please include $3.00 for postage and handling of books, $6 for international orders.

A complete catalogue of all book titles, audio lectures and courses, and videos is available upon request.

Visit us on the Internet at *http://www.som.org*